HAPPY LAND

ALSO BY DOLEN PERKINS-VALDEZ

Wench

Balm

Take My Hand

HAPPY LAND

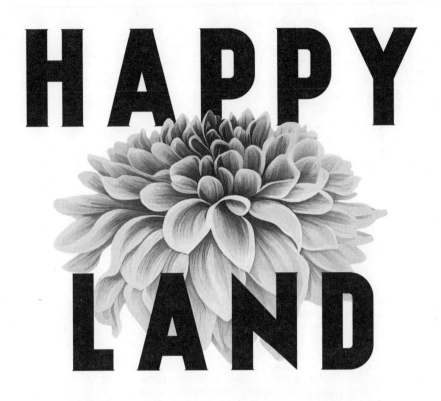

DOLEN PERKINS-VALDEZ

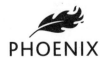

PHOENIX

First published in the United States in 2025 by Berkley
First published in Great Britain in 2025 by Phoenix Books,
an imprint of The Orion Publishing Group Ltd
Carmelite House, 50 Victoria Embankment
London EC4Y 0DZ

An Hachette UK Company

The authorised representative in the EEA is Hachette Ireland,
8 Castlecourt Centre, Dublin 15, D15 XTP3, Ireland
(email: info@hbgi.ie)

1 3 5 7 9 10 8 6 4 2

A CIP catalogue record for this book is
available from the British Library.

ISBN (Hardback) 978 1 4746 2271 4
ISBN (Export Trade Paperback) 978 1 4746 2272 1
ISBN (Ebook) 978 1 4746 2274 5
ISBN (Audio) 978 1 3996 2014 7

Printed and bound in Great Britain by Clays Ltd, Elcograf S.p.A.

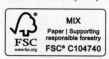

www.orionbooks.co.uk
www.phoenix-books.co.uk

Dedicated to my beloved sister. A queen among queens.
Jeanna McClure
1962–2021

OUR LAND

We should have a land of sun,
Of gorgeous sun,
And a land of fragrant water
Where the twilight is a soft bandanna handkerchief
Of rose and gold,
And not this land
Where life is cold.

We should have a land of trees,
Of tall thick trees,
Bowed down with chattering parrots
Brilliant as the day,
And not this land where birds are gray.

Ah, we should have a land of joy,
Of love and joy and wine and song,
And not this land where joy is wrong.

LANGSTON HUGHES

PART

ONE

ONE

Nikki

The only thing I know about my grandmother's home is that it's in an isolated area of the Blue Ridge Mountains in Zirconia, North Carolina. And the only thing I know about Zirconia is that it's right outside Hendersonville. And what I know about Hendersonville is that it has a lot of apple orchards.

A shame, I know.

The old 25 highway is two lanes without a line in the middle. I pass a wood-frame house that must be at least a hundred years old, a neat and tidy brick rambler with rockers lining the front porch. Stuffed fairies hang from tree limbs, and a motionless cat stares at me from a front yard.

I wind the rental car around a series of camp entrances. Camp Greystone. Camp Arrowhead. Houses on tall wooden piles perch around a sign labeled LAKE SUMMIT. Just a few miles past the lake, I pass the granite cliff Mother Rita mentioned over the phone, and just after that I reach the entrance to her property.

Lovejoy Lane.

When I was born, I was given my mama's maiden name hyphenated with Daddy's name—Lovejoy-Berry—in a gesture I'd always attributed to Mama's feminist pride. When I married Darius, I didn't change it. So seeing that Lovejoy sign does something to me. It looks official, as if the county provided it. I've never seen it before.

I'm almost forty years old, and this is my first time ever visiting my grandmother.

As I turn into the dirt drive I wonder how long my family has lived in this house. The siding is in need of a paint job, and the green shutters are faded and weather-beaten. I know Mama grew up here, and as I note its wide front porch and gabled roof, I imagine her, an only child, running down the front steps. It's morning, but the porch lamp is on, moth carcasses stuck to its dimly lit dome. I can't find a doorbell. I hesitate, then knock softly on the frame of the wooden screen door. A couple of minutes pass before I knock again.

Maybe she's asleep. The elderly do tend to keep their own hours.

Finally, the door opens and a tall lady with a shock of gray hair peers through the screen at me. "Yes?"

"Mother Rita?" I've always called her that, following Mama's lead.

"Veronica? I was expecting you later this evening."

"I'm sorry. They offered me a travel voucher, so I took a morning flight instead. I should have called."

"Yes, you should have." She pats her hair down.

Inside, the house is well kept—brighter and airier than I expected considering the condition of the exterior. Actually, I'm not sure what I expected, perhaps a dusty house filled with relics that

4

haven't been moved in years. Instead, the rooms are sunny, cheerful. I spy a settee too delicate for sitting in the living room, a tarnished silver tea set on a sideboard in the dining room, a Persian rug too big for the space. Everything is old, worn to the threads, but it's clean.

Mother Rita wears a pair of jeans and a neat, collared shirt turned up at the elbows. Despite her unruly hair, she looks pretty, especially for seventy-eight years old. It feels like forever since I've seen her. Actually, it's been eight years. I remember because when my daddy died, Mother Rita drove all the way to D.C. for the funeral, only to turn around and drive home the next day.

"You ate yet?"

"Yes, ma'am," I respond politely, though the truth is that I'm starving.

She glances down at the rolling suitcase I've just parked in the middle of her living room. It's as if she can see everything at once—my uncertainty, my curiosity, my fear.

"Bathroom is down the hall on the left. When you've finished, I got some leftover navy beans from yesterday. I'll warm those up with a little corn bread?" She uses a questioning tone, but I know there is no need to answer. This is her extension of hospitality, and I'm grateful for it.

A fuzzy pink rug covers the bathroom floor, its matching cover on the toilet seat. Behind the shower curtain, fish tiles rim the walls. Above the towel bar hangs a faded picture of a young man dangling a fish between his hands. My grandfather passed away when I was in elementary school. I lean closer to better make out his features.

I wash my hands slowly, taking my time. When Mother Rita called and asked me to come, the timing wasn't great. My daughter,

Shawnie, graduated high school last year and still doesn't have a full-time job. We've been fighting about it all summer. I've got a house on the market, but in the last couple of years I've lost my joy for selling real estate. I haven't sold a single property in months, and I'm about to run out of savings. If I don't get my act together, I'm going to be in real financial trouble soon. The truth of the matter is that my life is a mess right now.

When I hesitated, Mother Rita was insistent—*I need your help and if you come down here I will tell you everything your mama hasn't told you about our family.* It wasn't exactly an invitation I could refuse.

In the kitchen, she stands before the beans warming on the stove. I sit at the table, my eyes tracing her shoulders. I've seen Mother Rita only a handful of times in my entire life—my tenth birthday party at Crystal Skate, my high school graduation, Daddy's funeral. Even when Mother Rita did come to D.C., she and Mama were painstakingly polite, not like mother and daughter. I have always quietly believed they hated each other's guts, even before their final falling-out. All that to say that this is my first opportunity to spend time with my grandmother one-on-one without Mama's feelings running riot in the air. I want to ask her so many questions, but my tongue sticks to the roof of my mouth. Maybe after I get some food in my belly and we're seated across from one another, we can talk.

"You don't have a microwave?" I ask as she stirs.

"What's that, honey?"

"A microwave. To warm the beans."

"Oh, I don't fool with microwaves. Never have. Don't trust them."

I nod, wondering what other old notions she holds. I want to get up and help her, but she doesn't seem to invite the second pair of hands.

She spoons the beans into a bowl. "See, that didn't take long, did it? This fire suits me just fine."

"Smells good."

"I hope you don't mind the taste. I don't eat meat."

"I'll eat whatever is in that bowl," I say, though I am surprised to hear this. I wonder if she has always been vegetarian and if I just never realized it on those few occasions I've seen her. I know so little about this woman. My own kinfolk.

She slides a piece of foil out of the oven. The corn bread triangles are browned, edges crisped. She uses her bare fingers to drop the hot slices on the plate next to my bowl.

"Eat up. There's plenty," she says.

I want to talk more, but my stomach has other ideas. The beans aren't just salted. They contain something else that gives them depth, replacing the taste of a meaty bone.

"That's fresh fennel from my garden. I like to put it in my beans. Make a difference, don't it?"

My mouth is almost too full to respond. "It's really good. You ate already?"

"Don't worry about me none. There are more beans in the pot. Your room is the second door on the left. When you finish settling, come find me. I'll be in the yard out back."

I am awash in gratitude for this simple but hearty meal. I eat in silence after she leaves me.

I FINISH EATING and wash out my bowl before placing it in the empty dishwasher. Thank goodness my grandmother owns some of the other modern conveniences. The kitchen isn't large, but it's neat with an everything-in-its-proper-place kind of feel. A well-loved cast-iron skillet hangs from a nail on the wall. An old-fashioned bread box on the counter. A butcher's block of knives. The floor appears freshly swept. I am humbled by her tidiness, by the thought that this woman lives alone but keeps her house as if someone impressionable could drop by at any moment.

Or maybe I'm the impressionable person. Maybe she cleaned up knowing I was coming. The thought flushes me with unexpected warmth.

Mother Rita is an only child, Mama is an only child, I'm an only child, and so is my daughter, Shawnie. Granddaddy Herbert's people were from South Carolina, and he was a Jones, but Mother Rita kept the Lovejoy name and gave it to her daughter, an unusual choice for women of her generation.

I'd always wondered about that.

I know the Lovejoys have deep roots in the Hendersonville area, but beyond that I don't know much of the family history. Truth is, I've never been that interested in these mountains. Other than when Mama reminds me she was born and raised in Appalachia, I haven't thought about it much. To me, Appalachia is a concept. Something on television specials. Something I associate with old-time music.

But Mama's silence about her family has deepened my curiosity. She has rarely returned to North Carolina, and she never brought me or Shawnie with her. I'm curious how Mother Rita keeps herself entertained in this quiet neighborhood, living alone at her age. I hope things never get so bad between me and Shawnie that I end up alone.

I unpack in the small guest bedroom and go in search of her.

The coffeepot warmer is still on, and I stop to pour myself a cup. I need to call Shawnie and check on her, but before I do, I'd like to go to the supermarket. I want to get some things for Mother Rita, whatever she needs. I look around to see if there are other tasks needing to be done. The house is what we would call "cozy" in the real estate world. Just two bedrooms and a back sunroom that looks like an addition to the original house. For the first time, I see there isn't a leak or crack in the ceilings anywhere. The paint is fresh.

My grandmother has help. So why on earth does she need me?

"You like your room? I can't remember the last time I had a guest in there." Mother Rita appears in the doorway, a green scarf tied around her hair now. Her smooth brown skin is sun-kissed, eyes bright. She carries a basket with purple flowers hanging over the side.

"Was that Mama's room?"

"Course it was."

I'm surprised at the sudden coarseness of her tone. I don't remember her being sassy. "I love it, thank you. You've been outside?" I point down at her basket.

"Just picking a few wildflowers out back. Something about the way they follow their own mind out there makes me happy."

"I was thinking of finding somewhere in town for dinner. I want to treat you tonight."

"Oh, I don't really go out to eat these days. There used to be a place I liked in Hendersonville when my Herbert was alive. But they closed down, I heard." Her voice trails off.

"Okay."

"I do like to cook, though. Ain't no meal like the one in your own kitchen."

"Sounds good to me." I watch as she fills a vase with flowers. "What do you usually eat for dinner?"

"Sometimes I eat with my neighbor Maddie Mae. She has a grandson, and she cooks for him. If I don't feel like cooking, I call her up. But it's more likely I have something here. I've got a decent garden that push something out all year long. And I love fresh bread. You like bread or you one of them low-carb people?"

"No. I mean, yes. I love bread."

She smiles at me. "You're looking at me kind of funny. I like being out here, Veronica. I enjoy my peace and quiet. This is my home, the home of my ancestors. Our ancestors."

I put my cup down. "I still go by Nikki," I say, remembering that I've always had to correct her about my preferred name.

She blinks at me as if hearing this for the first time.

I don't want to appear rude, but I only have a week with her and I've got questions. Being here, it feels urgent, suddenly, that I know what happened that day she and Mama exchanged words for the last time. Long ago, I left them to stew in their corners, but since I'm here I may as well smoke Mother Rita out of hers.

I look her right in the eyes. "Mother Rita, why did you call me down here so suddenly? Are you going to tell me what happened between you and Mama?"

She fiddles with the flowers for a moment, as if trying to think of how to answer.

"There's time enough for that, Veronica. You'll know everything in due time, I promise."

"It's Nikki," I say softly, but she's already walking away.

TWO

Mother Rita asks a lot of questions. She knows I have questions of my own, but she seems determined to have hers answered first. *Is Lorelle dating anybody? Is she still in that same house in Michigan Park? Did she retire yet?* From the sound of it, Mother Rita misses Mama. She's just too stubborn to call her up and ask these questions directly.

We're sitting at the kitchen table. "What's our plan today?" I ask. "You need to go somewhere?"

"No, I got to do some cleaning up outside," she says. "Flower market is on Thursday."

"Flower market? You planning to buy some flowers?"

"Child, what kind of question is that? I'll show you my garden."

"I'd like that," I say. "Since you don't want to go out, I'll cook dinner tonight. Anything we can make out of your garden?"

"I do have a taste for some collards. There's a stockpot underneath that cabinet right there." She points.

"Alright," I say. We sit for a moment, the silence hanging between us awkwardly.

Mother Rita gets up from her chair. "Do you like to read?"

The question comes out of nowhere. "Y-yes. Sure I do."

"Oh yeah? What's the last book you read?"

I pause, trying to remember.

"You should read more," she says.

"It takes time to read, Mother Rita. I work a lot. D.C. is kind of a busy place to live."

"Don't act like D.C. is someplace special," she snaps. "I'm just as busy as you, and I still find time to read nearly fifty books a year. I didn't go to college, but I dare anybody to put a degree up against this." She taps her temple and I nod slowly.

Mother Rita is definitely saucier than I remember. And I'm stunned to learn that she reads so much. None of us went to college. Mama left North Carolina at eighteen and married my daddy a year later. I got married at nineteen just like her and studied to become a real estate agent. I'm still hoping Shawnie will take classes at the local college. At least she isn't married yet. That's progress.

She places a plastic library card in front of me. "This is my extra. While you're here, you can use it. Now, what kind of books do you like?"

I hesitate. "Mother Rita, I can't remember the last time I finished a book." Maybe it's my imagination but her face sags a little when I say that, so I add, "But I'll read anything you recommend." If reading a book or two helps me get closer to my grandmother, I'm willing to do it.

"You like history?" she asks.

I nod, though I prefer my history in movies.

"Alright." Mother Rita leaves the room and returns with a hardcover book.

"What's this?"

"It's a local history book. It tells all about the history of Henderson County. Maybe it'll teach you something about your roots."

I leaf through the book, looking for pictures. There aren't any.

"Did your mama ever tell you about the Kingdom of the Happy Land?" she asks.

"Kingdom of the what?"

"It was a community our people created after slavery times ended. I live on that land."

"No, Mama never told me anything about that," I say. "You're saying you live on land that used to be called a kingdom."

"Not called a kingdom. It was one."

"Oh, you're talking about a fiction novel?"

"No, Veronica. The kingdom was as real as the chair you're sitting in. And it was ruled by a king and queen, too."

I look at her incredulously, but Mother Rita sets me straight with her face. "Your ancestors lived here. Our ancestors," she adds.

I try not to sound disrespectful, but I still suspect she's exaggerating. "The next thing you'll be telling me is that your grandmother and granddaddy were the king and queen."

"My great-grandmother," she corrects. She isn't smiling, so I look down at the book, turning carefully back to the first page.

"Your great-grandmother and great-grandfather were the king and queen," I repeat and shake my head. "Of a real-life kingdom in North Carolina? How's that possible?"

"The locals around here like to say there weren't but two kingdoms in the history of the United States. This one and the kingdom of Hawaii," she says. "But that's not quite right because I've read about the kingdom of Hawaii. It was actually a sovereign state that was overthrown by the United States government."

My chin drops as if she's talking about ghosts and fairies, but I don't want to offend her any more than I already have. Finally, I say, "And this book tells about it?"

"Not a whole lot, but it's a start."

"What are you saying? And why hasn't Mama ever told me about this? She knows about it, too?"

She speaks so softly I can barely hear her. "I know you have questions, and I intend to answer them. I'm so glad you came, Veronica. Come on. Put your boots on and follow me out back. I want to show you something."

I wiggle my toes in my sandals. "I didn't bring boots, Mother Rita. It's summer."

"Boots aren't just for winter, child. It can get wet out there, especially after a rain. You bring any kind of real shoes?"

I know what she means—shoes that can get a little dirty, shoes that grip the ground so I won't slip and fall, closed-toe shoes to ward off a snakebite.

"What size are you?" she asks.

"Seven and a half."

"I think my neighbor who lives down the road wears your size. She probably got an extra pair. I need to give back her casserole dish anyway."

After she goes to her room to make the call, I pick up my phone, searching for "Kingdom of the Happy Land." There are only a few hits, so I quickly scan the articles. *A Black Kingdom in Postbellum Appalachia. Henderson County's Storied Kingdom.* Outside the window, the sky beckons and I'm more curious than ever to go out and see this fairy-tale land for myself. Surely it has to be special to inspire such tall tales.

After the borrowed boots appear on the doorstep, I follow Mother Rita out the back door. She lets the screen door slam behind us and doesn't lock it, grabbing a walking stick on the way out. I gather my braids into a bun and tie them on top of my head.

"Mother Rita, you lived in this house from what age?"

She looks back at me sharply, a crease across her face as she pulls a wide-brimmed hat down over her eyes. "My husband and his brothers built this house when I was a young bride. But my parents had a house about two hundred yards that-a-way. It's gone now."

The land stretches in all directions, but Mother Rita walks toward a line of trees that edges the field to what I believe is south. A trio of geese glides across the sky in a V formation, honking loudly. My mama can name a lot of birds by listening, and from a young age, she taught me some of the common birdsongs we hear in D.C. all the time. The first one I learned was the chipping of baby sparrows that would wake me up every spring. Being outside with Mama was understanding that we lived in a world of chatter, whether it be the *hoo* of the mourning doves that liked to nest in the eaves of our house or the clear whistles of robins that hopped through the yard. I'd always associated Mama's birdlove with her growing up in the country, but now I am standing in the very place she learned it.

"We going to see the garden?" I look off to my left where I glimpse rows of flowers surrounded by a fence made out of vertical wooden posts connected by wire netting. But Mother Rita is walking in another direction.

"Not yet. First, I want to show you something," she calls over her shoulder.

Seventy-eight years old and she can outwalk me. When we reach the line of trees, she uses her stick to beat back the brush, beckoning for me to follow. Finally, she stops at a small clearing and points to several mounds of carefully stacked rocks around the base of a tree.

I've seen these kinds of stacked rocks in a movie once. I think they're tributes to the dead. Did Mother Rita stack these rocks or did someone else? They look old and worn.

"What are these, Mother Rita?" I ask.

"These are my parents."

I squat to look. "What do you mean? Tributes to your parents? Or are they buried—"

"Yes, this is where they're buried."

I stand up and take a few steps back, suddenly afraid I'm standing right on top of their graves. There's no tombstone, no etching of names. Nothing. Sparse shoots of grass have long ago grown over the dirt.

"Mother Rita, why not put a headstone here? Somebody could cut down these trees and build something right over top of them."

"I won't allow it."

"You own all this land?"

I look back toward her house, nearly invisible in the distance. It's a lot of land—acres and acres of it.

"I used to bring your mama here, but she never showed any interest. I hope you'll be different." She gives me a look of disgust.

I don't know how to respond to that, and I don't like her saying negative things about Mama to me. "What happened between y'all, Mother Rita? What was so bad that—?"

"Pssh . . ." She makes a violent hushing noise that halts the words on my tongue. I frown. I'm starting to understand my mama's frustration with her. Conversations seem to be on Mother Rita's terms.

I look around. There are mounds of rocks everywhere I turn. "Mother Rita, what is this place?"

"Babygirl, this is your family graveyard. And one day I want you to bury me in it."

THREE

Luella

The farm in South Carolina was known as Lily of the Valley, though none of us had ever known such a flower and we sure wasn't in no valley. That was just what they called the place, a home filled with the most beautiful furniture you ever seen. We was owned by a white man by the name of Bobo. To say that he did not kill us was to give him a compliment of sorts.

By the time I was born in 1850, Mister Bobo was at the height of his powers, his two-hundred-acre farm rich with corn and wheat. In the quarters, there was a blacksmith shop, a barn, a meat house, a well house with cellar, and a kitchen. The man never allowed us to go hungry, and I guess that was a compliment of sorts, too.

I worked in the house and was raised alongside his daughter, though I was not allowed to touch the books that lined Mister Bobo's library. In them days, I thought books was magical, that they cast spells. To read was to have the language to ask for the things you wanted, so I became determined to teach myself.

My papa was a minister to us in slavery, and after it ended, he became a minister to us in freedom. Papa stood erect, with a high chin and broad flat forehead, skin as dark as shoe leather, and legs that moved gracefully, like the strides of a bird.

Papa kept me close, having lost my mother in the birthing of me, their only child. I was valued for my sewing skills, though I never enjoyed the task. I had been taught by a trio of women who took me, a motherless girl, under their care.

After freedom, we settled in nearby Cross Anchor, not far from the old plantation farm, where Papa built a church on a piece of land rented from the man who owned the town store. Others who'd worked the iron mills up in Spartanburg moved down our way, some to escape trouble. Our names was few—Casey, Whitmire, Bobo, Bennett, Sheldon, Couch—and though some chose a new name right off, most of us kept the names of our white folk.

I was twenty years old when the Montgomery brothers joined Papa's church. They had been part of the Montgomery plantation, a little-known place where it was whispered the owners raised children to sell. They kept to themselves before freedom, so we hadn't seen their people much. But from the time the brothers joined the church, they caught the eyes of the women.

Both of the brothers was tall, tall as I'd ever seen on a man. Both was thin, with bodies as willowy as branches. The older one had a square chin and a straight mouth that didn't move much when he formed words, though when he spoke, people seemed to listen. The younger one had a rounder face, and though he was a little shorter than the other, he was still tall as a weed. The younger brother had a hearty laugh, and on more than one occasion I heard him before I saw him. Once, he caught me looking and smiled the broadest smile. I was carrying a cake made by one of the church members and I nearly dropped it.

Later that night, Jola Casey and me was cleaning up the dishes, wiping out plates and emptying cups. The two of us had been sharing secrets since we was girls, so I leaned forward to listen when she said, "He asking about you."

"Who?" I said.

"The tall one."

I shook my head. Surely she was mistaken. It was the younger brother who had smiled at me. And wasn't they both tall? "You sure it was the older one?"

She nodded. "I heard him asking about you."

I knew I was what men considered pretty. From a young age, I had understood I possessed a value that could be counted in coins but also in pleasure. My hair was thick, and it grew long without much attention. I kept it in a braid wrapped around my head. On Sundays I walked down to the creek, let my hair down, and washed it in the water. Everybody said I looked like my mama, though I had no memory of her face.

My papa swore an oath to protect me from white men when we was enslaved. One look in his eye, and everybody could see he would die for that oath. Now this Montgomery brother was asking after me, and I was at an age when Papa might agree to a suitor he liked.

Jola had always been more the type to fight with boys than kiss them. Once, when one of them pulled her hair, she punched him right in the eye with her fist. She had been known to pass off boys to me, and I thought maybe she was doing it this time, too.

"How do you know he asking about me? Maybe he asking about you."

She giggled and pulled playfully at my braid. "Do I got long hair? That's what he said. *Who the girl with all the hair?*"

When I returned home that night, to the two rooms I shared with Papa that he'd built behind the church, the Montgomery brother was standing outside. He reached out a hand, as if to shake mine. I didn't take it. "My name William," he said.

Up close, I could see he was older than I was, not gray hair old but the mature face of a man who had seen his share of sunrises. There was a light in his eye that caught my attention, something I couldn't turn away from.

"My papa call me Lu," I said, and for some reason I kept talking. "But you can call me Luella."

He smiled. "Nice to meet you, Miss Luella."

And I allowed William Montgomery to take my hand in his for the first time.

THE KU KLUX Klan rose up in Spartanburg County after the war ended, and they was so awful that U.S. president Grant got involved. They had been beating on us and murdering us ever since we was freed, but it got worse after we started voting. Next thing they know we was in the statehouse and even elected a colored state secretary. The more we used our vote, the worse it got, so we didn't dare go out after dark. Some of us even kept a rifle under the bed, though to use it was death, too.

In 1870, the federal soldiers came down to our state and started arresting Klansmen left and right. Everybody was scared, even the bravest among us. You would think the presence of them federal soldiers would make us feel safe, but we knew if the white South Carolinians was in trouble, so was we. So we stepped careful and tried to go about our days.

The Klansmen trials started in the fall of 1871 when I was

twenty-one years old. Papa's church held news sessions every Wednesday night. Us ones that knew our letters got hold of the paper and read to us that couldn't. We only lit enough candles to see the paper, the rest of us in darkness so the gatherings wouldn't attract attention. Week after week, we heard the convictions coming through. We knew they couldn't get them all but maybe they could get the worst ones. At least, that's what we hoped. Course we knew better than to trust the punishment would fit the crimes.

Meanwhile, the statewide elections was coming up again, and Papa helped register more voters. During our Wednesday news sessions, we discussed colored candidates for state office, and though the women couldn't cast a ballot, we didn't hold back our opinions. The church was more than a place for the holy spirit; it was also a place for politics.

The federal government ended the trials in early 1873, and things in Cross Anchor quieted. We wasn't being attacked as often, but the whole town felt like it was sitting on a powder keg. Then Papa got picked up by the law and carried down to the center of town where they'd built a whipping post. He yelled at me not to follow, but I refused to let them do it without the burn of my eyes on their backs. If they was going to whip my Papa, they was going to have to do it in front of God and his daughter.

I knew why they'd picked him out. Papa wasn't just voting, though that was reason number one. Most of the colored men in the county was voting, and with Papa encouraging them, that was reason enough, too. Before freedom, we'd been members of the white church, where we sat in the back and listened to how we was the sons of Ham and bore the mark of Cain. Now we made our own stories from the Bible, and white people was mighty scared of a colored preacher spinning tales they couldn't control, especially when them stories gave us wings.

But I believed Papa's prosperity was another reason they came for him. His crops was getting to be valued at over eight hundred dollars each year. That was more than most coloreds and even some white men earned. It was a wonder they didn't kill my papa, though that was right around the time we started thinking they might. When the whipping was over, I took Papa's arm and helped him stand up straight as we walked back home, and for three days I didn't leave his side.

Just weeks after the public whipping, Harry Norman stopped by to deliver news that shook Papa even more. A journalist had written something about our congregation in the *Carolina Spartan* that told a lie too strange to believe.

ZION'S TRAVELERS

A MURDEROUS RELIGIOUS ORGANIZATION OF BLACKS

WORSE THAN VOODOO

They accused us of holding an elderly woman hostage while planning to sacrifice her. They even said we planned to eat her! They wrote that Papa was evil and held us in a spell.

The white owner of the store—and our land—gave the warning. There was trouble afoot, the man told Papa, and he would release him from his debt if he decided to leave town. *That's awful nice of you*, Papa said, watching him closely.

That evening, when I returned to the house, Papa was waiting for me. He called me to have a seat, and what he said next shocked me breathless.

"What if I told you we might need to leave Cross Anchor."

"What you mean leave Cross Anchor?" I was confused by his use of the phrase *what if*.

"It ain't safe around here, and William been telling me—"

"William?"

He nodded. "William Montgomery been telling me about a place up in the hills where we can find work. I was going to talk to the church about it, see what people think. It's bad here, Lu. The man at the store say trouble brewing."

"What kind of trouble?"

"What other kind is there."

Course what Papa meant was that this was a trouble we might not survive, something bad enough to not just threaten our livelihoods, but our lives. Still, Cross Anchor was our home.

"But they put the Klansmen in jail. They had trials," I said.

"You know well as I do this still Klan country."

I wondered if this was William's idea, if he had convinced Papa of some imaginary land of milk and honey. Papa was being too trusting of this man.

"Lu, I won't make this decision without your approval. What do you think we should do?"

One thing was true. That newspaper article wasn't good in no way whatsoever. But at least here in this little town, it was a devil we knew. I wanted to say all these things, but Papa was asking my thoughts and I wanted to prove I could handle his confidence. So I nodded and took his hand.

"Course I'm with you, Papa. Whatever you need me to do, just let me know."

He smiled and closed his eyes, gripping my fingers in his.

That night Papa called a church meeting.

We met in the sanctuary, and he shared with the congregation what the store owner had told him. There arose a clamor so loud even Papa had trouble settling it. Finally, the congregation hushed, waiting expectantly for what their pastor would say next. The white folk in town was right about one thing. Papa held power among his people, respect, though he never asked nobody to do nothing against their wishes.

"They ain't gone stop till they destroy us. We ain't got no choice but to leave. Sell what you can over the next day or so and, on the third day, we set out," Papa said as a groan arose from the group.

Where we going? they asked.

He raised his hands. "Now, you can stay if you want. I ain't forcing nobody to do nothing. But I'm going."

Where we going? they repeated.

William Montgomery stood up. Papa's church had room for about five dozen people on the wooden benches. Lit candles lined the walls, and the flickering light cast shadows on our faces. He spoke quietly, told us of this place he knew at the top of the mountain just over the state line, a place where we could be safe and live free from the terror of the Klan. His words enticed us, and I'd be lying if I said I didn't fall under the spell, too.

We was so quiet as he spoke, sharing this vision. Quiet as church mice. Quiet as sleeping babies deep in dreamland.

TO GO NORTH, even if it was only for sixty or so miles, was to leave behind everything we had built. In our haste, we sold our livestock for less than it was worth—cows for as low as a dollar and a half, hogs for as low as a dollar. Papa sold five hundred dollars' worth of crops for just one hundred. We packed as much as we could sensibly carry, but it was inevitable some had to leave behind chairs they'd made from raw wood, bedding they'd sewn from scrap cloth, pots and pans bartered with small jobs.

And then there was our houses. Some of us lived in old quarters, but the most prosperous of us had built wooden houses from the ground up. Even if the land was rented, we was allowed to build our homes, and we took pride in the structures. Them little houses might have been the most painful things to bid farewell.

Just days after that nighttime meeting, we was on our way.

We didn't have no map or compass that might help guide us. We headed north the way people before us had done it, following memory.

I ain't never met a road that traveled in a circle, William said when somebody doubted him.

He became our leader, moving ahead to spur us on, for the hill we climbed was steep. The Montgomery brothers had traveled the Buncombe Turnpike before. Back when they belonged to Mister Montgomery, they'd transported cargo back and forth, and been hired out for animal husbandry.

We moved slow, some of the women carrying children and babies on their backs. The elderly stopped to rest. The healthy held the hands of the sick. At night, we slept on the ground, rolls of clothes beneath our heads. Papa must have been more tired than I was, but he never showed it. Even when I woke before him, it only took a light touch before his eyes opened and he gathered himself.

There was close to fifty of us—men, women, and children. As we climbed the mountain, a few decided to turn back. I kept my eyes on Papa, who gave his blessing at sunrise each morning.

Jola traveled with her parents and younger brother. When her brother tired, her papa carried him, and when her papa tired, Jola took over. At night, I gave Jola my blanket as she rested for the next day's journey.

The air thinned as we walked, my throat wanting more water than was rationed. All around us there was mountain wilderness, and I had never seen such land. Cross Anchor had been flat and wide. This land was hilly and green. The road curved like a snake, and with each turn I fretted we wouldn't make it.

One day William handed me his canteen. "Drink," he said.

I gulped and he didn't slow me. Finally, I tried to give it back to him. "I didn't mean to drink so much. I was thirsty."

He pushed the canteen back to me. "Drink it all. I fill it up again at the next watering hole."

I shook my head. He was leading the group, walking the fastest.

"Drink," he said again. I finished it off and thanked him. I could feel the other women watching as he walked away.

Finally, we came upon the sign for an inn that read OAKLAND. A white woman in a dark mourning dress came outside and stood a ways off from us, quietly observing. We must have looked ragged and hungry, because she did not make eye contact with nobody other than William. He called her Missus Davis, and I knew I wasn't the only one among us who wondered if she would refuse him and send us on our way.

After speaking quietly with the woman, William returned to where our group was sitting under the shade of a maple tree. We would work at the inn and tend her land, settling in the old slave quarters she still owned. It wasn't clear at first what kind of labor she required, but we was prepared for most everything. We wasn't no stranger to the field or the house.

"Who is she?" somebody asked after William was finished talking.

"That's the Widow Davis," he answered and motioned for us to follow him back across the turnpike.

FOUR

The first thing the men did was repair the roof of the inn. They started by patching the holes that allowed the rain inside. They filled ceiling cracks and painted walls and fixed broken furniture. Nails poked up out of the wooden floors, and the men took hammers to them. The Cross Anchor women shook carpets, swept under beds, and dusted windowsills. We took down curtains, washing and ironing before hanging them again. We emptied out closets, raked flower beds, washed windows.

Since her husband died, the most the Widow had been able to manage was a cook who handled everything from meals to laundry and a second woman who made beds and emptied bedpans. Them two was more than glad to see us arrive.

Some of us was accustomed to a house as grand as the Lily of the Valley, so the Widow's inn was nothing. Her location on the turnpike was a good one; if we got the house in order, we would prove to be worth the trouble.

The Widow kept us busy. Though she hoped for fall and winter visitors, there was too much work to be done. So we prepared for when the low-country travelers would make their way up the mountain for cooler weather in the summer. The rumor was that she had already raised her nightly lodging price, the first increase since the war. She was trying to attract the best travelers again, and she knew our help would make the difference.

Our people worked hard to be useful, to make our arrangement with the Widow last. Some of the men hunted, bringing her freshly killed duck and wild turkey. Come springtime, when most of the work on the inn would probably come to an end, we decided we would plant crops and supply her with food.

In return, the Widow allowed us to move into the two dozen slave cabins that remained from before the war. She owned so much land that the old quarters was about a mile from the inn. That meant there was quite a bit of timber, so we began to build more houses in the manner we had in Cross Anchor. Our houses back home had been two and three rooms, so while we stayed in the Widow's one-room cabins, the men began to see to larger ones for families.

We considered sunlight and the slope of the land. Would water flow away when it rained. Would the light hit the garden at the right time of day. We laid out the basic plan of the settlement, altered what had already been there when we arrived. If anyone raided us they would have to get past a dozen houses to reach our stores. That was William's plan, and it was a good one.

At our entrance, we built a fence between two trees and somebody painted PRIVAT on it. One of the children wrote out the letters, and for weeks to come I would walk past the sign and stop to say each letter separately.

P-R-I-V-A-T.

Cutting down trees took time. A straight trunk was best. There wasn't no horses to haul logs so the men carried them, sometimes five men hefting a large one. They etched the notches in careful round scoops and stacked them to create walls.

I delighted in seeing the four walls go up. Children gathered stones from the Green River, and we set the corners for fireplaces. The women mixed dirt and water to fill the gaps. We carved out windows, then covered them with greased paper. When the roof went on, we ended the day with cheers of jubilation.

P-R-I-V-A-T.

There had been no walls in slavery times. There had been no assumption that somebody might want to eat and sleep in two different rooms. Many of us had lived in nothing bigger than a twelve-foot square, so we put up them walls with the kind of joy that only a person who has been treated less than human can understand.

Working together was exactly the balm our souls needed in them early months. At night some of us shared stories, unloading what we had brought up the mountain on our backs. Others merely listened, determined to keep their hurt bottled up. Some of our people wanted to go back to South Carolina. It had been our home, after all. But we couldn't go back. The lie they'd told about us still rang loudly in our ears. Somebody had gotten their hands on a New York newspaper. For some reason, the lie was being printed far and wide. After word got out about us heading north, it was as if they spit on the trail we left behind. Papa believed we got out in the nick of time.

One evening after dinner, just before sunset, a meeting for every member of the community was called. We'd built up the settlement so that it encircled a central tree—a massive oak with gnarled branches that the children loved to climb. We sat on the grass, some of us rolling out pallets. A few of the men fashioned rudimentary sitting posts for the elders. We had been in North Carolina for nearly three months, and we was expecting one of our men, Reverend Couch, to return any day with at least a dozen more people.

William was the only one standing, his brother, Robert, sitting attentively at his feet.

"Good evening," William began. "I hope y'all don't mind me calling this meeting. We been here for a while now, but we been so busy working, we ain't stopped to rest much."

We turned our attention to him. We numbered over forty, so quieting us was no small feat.

"I called y'all here because I got something to say, something to . . . suggest." He said the word as if it was one he had considered beforehand. "I don't see no reason for us to run this place like how we lived back in Cross Anchor. We get to make our own rules now."

Suggest. What a pretty word. I could barely follow because I was busy turning the sound of it over in my head.

"What you talking about, William?" Hal Whitmire asked.

"Me and my brother, Robert, we knew our daddy and our daddy's daddy. They had memories of the home place, and back over there, our people was royalty. They ruled a kingdom. We here on this mountain, in these woods, away from the white man's government. We make our own government, our own rules. We need to make this place like Africa."

Africa! Laughter arose among us.

Did he say Africa?

Sure did.

William ignored the chatter. "First, we need a ruling council—a group of men to settle disputes, make laws."

Hal shook his head. "A council, huh? I don't know, William. Ain't no place in this country the white man's laws can't reach. If you saying we make our own country, the South tried to do that during the war, and it's a lot of them rolling around in their graves 'cause of it."

"I'm not talking about a country," William responded. "I'm talking about a kingdom."

We rustled, looked around in confusion. But my papa didn't move, not one inch. He was all ears.

William kept on. "I'm just saying the Widow got a lot of land here. And she can't handle it alone, not without our help. But we can make our own place on it. Our own rules. A kingdom like what we ruled back in the home place."

"What you talking about? We up here starting from nothing. I sold everything I owned to come up that hill," Hal bellowed.

"Look, Hal!" William pointed into the distance. "That turn-pike got travelers on it. Just like the Widow getting money, we can, too."

What he talking about money? More rumblings.

"Second thing. We need a treasury."

"Treasure? Like gold?" somebody shouted.

"Treasury. A place for our earnings."

I thought of the cloth pouch where I'd kept Papa's coins back in Cross Anchor. I had been his treasury. I'd never heard this word before, but it felt nice on my lips. William was sharp as a knife, I was realizing.

"Everything we earn, we need to put in the kingdom treasury. Don't we got more if we put it all together?"

Everybody began to murmur in agreement, even the women. We knew the power of money even if most of us had never held a paper note in our hands. But I had just heard William use the word *kingdom* for the third time, and I was still confused by what he meant.

"Right now we working for the Widow to get the inn back up and running. But I hear tell there's work nearby. Blacksmithing work. Horseshoeing. Carpentry. I know a lot of y'all can earn something round here. We buy our own seed, plant our own crops. Get the things we need."

Our people in Cross Anchor had been skilled, so we knew we could do what he was asking.

"What about voting?" Hal Whitmire asked.

"We leave it behind," William said sharply. "We make our own laws up here."

Not vote? Just the thought scared me. Voting was what it meant to be a citizen, a generational wish passed down from our parents and grandparents. It had been the laws that had enslaved us in the first place. Only way to change the law was to vote. Could we really escape this country and all its disorder up here on this mountain?

William's younger brother turned to the group. "I agree with my brother. We can make a life here. And why can't we work hard and even buy this land one day? We already tried voting and look where it got us. They killed us for it. It's better to own land."

Now you could hear a fly buzz. Nobody said a word at that. I stared at Robert, curious. How did he expect us to buy land?

John Earl Casey, Jola's daddy, chimed in quietly, his voice shaking with emotion. "The Klan killed my pa for voting. He was eighty-three years old. Eighty-three! I ain't going back. You tell me how to make a life here for my family and I'll make it out of nothing with my own two hands."

Papa stood. "I'm with you, William. I'll help set up the council."

We got real quiet at that, because while William was taking charge, we trusted Papa. He was our spiritual leader.

Margaret Couch spoke from her position on top of a blanket. "Whatever the men need, the womenfolk will help," she said. "But tell me, William. What you mean by kingdom?"

At first, William didn't answer. As I watched the men and women around us digest his dream, his vision for us, I could see that he had inspired belief in the same way he had sold us on the idea of making this trip in the first place.

With his words.

"I'm saying we make this place a kingdom, just like back in Africa. I'm saying we need to claim our royal robes." His voice boomed in the clearing.

It would be a few more weeks before the council gathered for the first time. But that night William Montgomery planted the seed. And it was a seed that would grow.

FIVE

Nikki

All my life I've been part of a small family circle. By the time my daddy was twenty, both of his parents had passed away. He and Mama, with their desire to build a family out of nothing, were a perfect match for each other in that way. The two of them against the world. For me, not having a sibling or even a cousin has been the only existence I've ever known. Now here I am walking beside my grandmother on acres and acres of land that my people have inhabited for over a hundred years. It's hard to put how I'm feeling into words other than to say I'm dizzy with grief. I didn't know you could mourn something you never had.

On our way back to the house, we stop at the gardens. Beyond the gate, a whole world awaits. This is no mere hobbyist's spread. The plantings are separated by mulched paths about three feet wide, and the rows teem with color. I wander among them, trying to pick out what I recognize before looking down to read the small signs staked into the dirt. Delphiniums tower over zinnias. A patch of snapdragons next to impossibly tall sunflowers. Rows of foxglove and lavender. At the end, there's a cedar bench. I imagine Mother Rita sitting on it with a book.

Surely Mother Rita doesn't tend to all this by herself. It's like a small farm.

She's watching me, so I say, "This is all yours?"

"Everything in it." She walks over to a delicate flower with a blossom as big as my face. "You ever seen a dinnerplate dahlia? These are my girls."

I can't help noticing that she talks about the flowers with more affection than she speaks of us, her actual girls. It's a weird kind of jealousy, but I feel it just the same.

"My mama and daddy farmed this land. When they got too old to work it, we hired out some hands to help. Those fields are long gone now. I just grow flowers these days."

"This is a lot, Mother Rita."

"How do you think I support myself?"

"I never knew you made a living with flowers." I'd always assumed my granddaddy Herbert was the breadwinner. He worked at the General Electric plant for years. I figured Mother Rita lived. off his retirement after he passed away, but now I remember just how long he's been gone.

"I do pretty good during wedding season. I sure am glad you're here to help. Usually, Maddie Mae and her son help me."

We walk along the path that cuts through the plantings. In the supermarket where I shop, most flowers come in anonymous bunches, and I know the usuals—roses, chrysanthemums, daisies, peonies, tulips. But there is abundance here, flowers I can't name. "How do you decide what to grow?"

"Most important for me is vase life. You don't want folk buying your flowers at market only to have them die in a few days. I love zinnias for this reason. They can last a while plus they come in a lot of colors."

I lean to sniff one of the bright ones.

"Aren't you precious. Sorry to tell you zinnias don't smell like nothing. The snapdragons smell nice, though." She continues walking. "Second, they got to be hardy. We cut and transport and make bouquets. So you don't want a flower so delicate it falls apart before somebody can get it home. These cosmos are good for that. And those black-eyed Susans over there."

"Sounds complicated."

"Oh, child, it's easy. You could learn it if you wanted. I do believe this garden has added years to my life."

We pause, and she turns her face into the sun. I can now see that it's a gardener's face. Or at least what I imagine one might look like. Weathered, but peaceful. This is where Mother Rita belongs. She'd wilt in a city like D.C. even if she could visit the National Arboretum every day. Out here on this mountain where neighbors are too far to be heard and the worst threat to mammals is the crack of a rifle, she floats. There is an undeniable contentment to her. I'd always pictured Mother Rita distraught over her lack of close family, but now I wonder if she even cares that she barely knows me. My heart clouds with the thought.

"My mama," I whisper, hesitantly, because I don't know what fire I might stir. "Did she grow up gardening with you?"

She turns to me and cocks her head to one side as if in confusion. "Of course she did. She worked in this very garden, on this very land. Didn't she teach you nothing at all about flowers?"

I shake my head. At Mama's house, we have azalea bushes and that's it. We don't even have indoor plants. Though Mama loves birding and taking walks outdoors, she never said anything about a garden. It's difficult to imagine her out here with dirty finger-nails. During the week, she dresses for her government accounting job, and on the weekends, she goes to dance class and volunteers at a local food bank.

Mother Rita squats and fingers the soil. I'm impressed at her agility. I don't have the knees for squatting. But Mother Rita seems comfortable, as if she could sit on her haunches all day long. She mumbles, but I can't hear what she's saying. It sounds disgruntled, but it also sounds like she's speaking to someone.

"Mother Rita?"

She stands and faces me. "It hurts my heart that your mother lost her way and kept you so far from your people. Come on. We don't have much time and I got a lot to teach you."

I follow her back to the house, my eyes wide as I realize she has just been talking to the flowers.

THAT EVENING, I wash the collards and cut them into ribbons. The skillet heats up, and I pour a dollop of oil before adding a heap of fresh garlic from her patch. Then I add the greens. After they've sauteed a few minutes, I add a little apple cider vinegar and vege-table broth.

I can't shake the image of that family graveyard. It seems a shame there are no names or dates of birth and death. I wonder how many Mother Rita can identify. She should add name plac-ards and fence it in so it won't ever be destroyed.

How could that be my family graveyard? Except for Grand-daddy Herbert's gravestone, it's nothing but piles of rocks. Mother Rita said her great-grandmother was the queen of this so-called kingdom. I wonder if she's buried there, too.

As the greens simmer, I sit in the kitchen chair scrolling on my phone for grave markers to price them out. The graves should be marked. Maybe I could sketch out a diagram and have Mother Rita write everything down before I leave in a few days. I can't believe I'm being drawn into a graveyard project when the only reason I came down here was to learn what caused this rift between Mama and Mother Rita and help her with whatever was so urgent. Now here I am looking up gravestones and acting like my family isn't a hot mess of secrets.

I go in search of Mother Rita and find her sitting in the chair in the back room. At first it appears she's nodding off, but as I draw closer I can see her eyes are wide open and she's staring out the window. I look to see what's out there, but all I can see is the great expanse of land underneath the late afternoon sun.

"Dinner's just about ready," I tell her.

"Smells good. I can't remember the last time somebody else cooked in my kitchen."

I decide to seat us at the formal dining table rather than in the kitchen. It's a little dim in there, and when I look up, I discover that one of the bulbs in her ceiling light is out. I'll pick up some lightbulbs on my trip to the store.

"I don't eat in the dining room much anymore. Not since my Herbert died."

"It's a special occasion," I say, trying to sound cheery. "I'm visiting my grandmother for the first time."

She follows me into the dining room and watches as I light two candles I found in her cupboard.

"It's a shame how your mama has treated me all these years, keeping y'all away from here."

"For what it's worth, Mama never said anything bad about you."

"I'm guessing she didn't say much about me at all."

It's true. Mama's response to my questions over the last several years has been an infuriating silence. I have even learned to anticipate the telltale set of her lip that happens whenever I bring up Mother Rita's name. "Only you and Mama know why that is."

"It's because she's a Judas, that's why."

I'm grown enough to know that both of them are being stubborn, but I still don't like her insulting Mama. "Mother Rita, what do you mean she's a Judas? Why won't you tell me why you and Mama don't talk anymore? What did she ever do to you?"

"Like you said, that's between me and her."

"That's not what I said. This is between all of us. I'm almost forty years old! Don't you think I deserve the truth?"

She purses her lips and folds her arms across her chest.

"Did this all start because Mama moved away? Because that was four decades ago. Get over it." I can scarcely believe I'm talking to her like this, and it looks like she can't believe it either, because she gives me a hard look that makes me want to go sit in a corner.

"I don't give a damn about her moving," she says. "Good riddance. I'm fine with or without her."

Mother Rita says this with the kind of passion that speaks the exact opposite of her words. Of course she cares Mama left. I know this feud didn't start with an argument eight years ago. The milk had been spoiled a long time before that. The contours of Mama's story ring in my head. Mama left for D.C. after high school. Granddaddy Herbert sent money, but only if Mama asked, and without Mother Rita's knowledge. Once Mama married Daddy, Mother Rita knew she'd never return to live in North Carolina and she'd taken the rejection personally. After Granddaddy Herbert died, she even blamed Mama for her loneliness.

I'm just so tired of carrying these grown women on my back. But I'm here now, and I am determined to get some answers.

After I serve our food, we eat quietly, and I sneak peeks at her—this regal woman who only eats vegetables and reads fifty books a year.

"Tell me more about the graveyard out back," I say to calm the air. "And the Kingdom of the Happy Land."

"I already told you. There was a queen and a king. They were your ancestors. You come from royalty."

It all sounds like one elaborate folktale to me, but I dare not say that. I am tiptoeing around her moods, and I don't want to flip the apple cart. "And this queen. What was her name?"

"Luella."

I repeat the name softly. *Luella.* "And she was African?"

She scowls at me. "Aren't we all?"

I nod slowly. Maybe Mother Rita is one of those people who believe all African Americans are African, not just descendants, as a way of more forcefully claiming our heritage.

She sighs, as if talking to a small child. "It'll take a while to piece it together, but I believe you can do it."

"Piece what together? Mother Rita, I leave on Sunday. I've got a listing, and I really need to sell this one. Otherwise, I'm not going to be able to pay—"

She gives a little shake of her head as if I've said nothing. "They were Montgomerys, Caseys, Whitmires, Bennetts. But she was born Luella Bobo on the Bobo plantation down in Cross Anchor, South Carolina. I want you to learn as much as you can about her because the story of this land is tied up with her."

"You mean the story about how that graveyard came to be out there?"

42

"Not just the graveyard. The land. She was powerful, a natural-born leader, according to my mama." She leans back in her chair.

"Maybe I'll come back sometime in the fall during the holidays. We can do some research."

"You come back in the fall and it'll be too late."

"Too late for what? And what exactly did you need my help with?"

"You said you want to know the truth about what happened between me and your mama, didn't you? It all starts with Luella."

"How could your feud with Mama start with a woman who lived over a hundred and fifty years ago? I mean, I get that she's our ancestor, but the past is past—"

"You sound just like Lorelle."

Her words silence my outburst. And they hurt. It's not just that she has compared me to Mama, it's that she has said it with such nastiness. I bite my lower lip, trying to hold back tears. I think about leaving early, changing my flight. I have a client waiting for me to sell their house, a monster of a rowhouse that is badly in need of a renovation and overpriced by at least thirty thousand. On top of that, my only child has shut down on me and seems to be heading nowhere fast.

I've wasted my time coming down here. She doesn't need me to help her with anything.

"Veronica, I'm sorry." She utters the words slowly, as if they pain her. I can tell she isn't used to apologizing. "I shouldn't have said that."

I shrug a little, as if to say it was no big deal, though I know that isn't true.

She bites into her corn bread.

My chest feels tight so I pretend to go back for seconds. In the

43

kitchen, I lean against the wall to steady myself. It's all too much to take. My great-great-great-grandmother was the self-anointed queen of some kind of remote Black community. There's a pile of rocks out back with a bunch of my ancestors buried under them. And I still don't know why the women in my family refuse to speak. I fill a glass with water from the tap and down it.

When I return to the dining room, I fumble my next question, speaking in a tiny voice. I didn't know this was a fear until I say it aloud. "Will you stop talking to me if I go back home, Mother Rita? Like when Mama left?"

Mother Rita stares at me for a minute, as if shocked by the question. Her words are kind, but her voice doesn't soften.

"You're a precious young lady and I so appreciate you. I wish we'd gotten to know each other sooner. I know this has got to be hard for you. Pour me some more of that tea, will you."

My hand shakes as I spill a little tea on her tablecloth, but she doesn't seem to notice.

SIX

The final split between Mama and Mother Rita happened not long after Daddy died.

My mama, an accountant for the Treasury Department for over thirty years, was—how do I put it—unraveled by my daddy's death. That's the best word I can use to describe it. Mama, who wore sensible pumps she purchased from one of those comfort shoe stores in Dupont Circle, who believed navy, brown, and gray were the only three colors suitable for work, who ironed pleats into the jeans she wore on weekends, began putting her shirts on backward, wearing scuffed Converse sneakers, and forgetting her second earring. She'd walk all the way to the Metro and forget her Metro Card. In supermarkets, she took the wrong cart and didn't realize it until she was in checkout. At night, I found the refrigerator door left open and once even discovered the unattended gas stove emitting a low blue flame.

My perfectionist, keep-it-all-together Mama was now a shell

of herself, and I watched as lines etched her face and gray hairs sprouted in her temples, as if in real time. Daddy's death aged Mama, and though I was just as bereft as she was, there was only space for her grief. It was as if I'd lost both my parents.

It was the year I turned twenty-eight. Shawnie was just starting third grade. When Daddy got sick, I passed my listings to another agent and helped Mama take care of him, Darius right beside me. Usually charismatic and outgoing, Darius was quiet and gentle with Daddy, helping to move him from his chair to the bed when he became too heavy for me and Mama. Though our marriage wasn't doing well at the time, Darius did not hesitate to step right up and show my daddy a tenderness he would have shown his own.

A few months after Daddy passed, Mama stopped by our apartment unexpectedly on a Saturday.

"Where's Darius and Shawnie?" she asked.

"They went to the park."

She poured a cup of coffee from the carafe on the counter. "This coffee's cold."

"It's been sitting there all day. You want me to warm it up?"

Sometimes I got my old mama, the one who used to write out weekly calendars on the refrigerator and planned vacations months in advance. Other times, the new mama appeared, disheveled, vacant. I didn't know until I'd lost it how much Mama's Virgo predictability had stitched our lives together. Darius was the answer to my grief. Mama didn't have an answer to hers.

"I've got something to tell you," she said.

"Okay." My mind went directly to the worst place. Please, Lord, don't let Mama be sick. I couldn't take that kind of news again. But what she said next puzzled me.

"Your grandmother isn't in our lives anymore."

"Mother Rita? What do you mean?"

Mama wouldn't make eye contact with me. She traced the rim of the mug with a finger, over and over.

"What do you mean? Did she—?"

"No, she's still in the land of the living, if that's what you're asking."

Mama sometimes used country sayings that reminded me she was from North Carolina.

"So what do you mean she's not in our lives?" She had just been in D.C. for the funeral, and though they'd acted in their typical frosty way, she'd stayed at Mama's house for one night.

"I just got off the phone with her. She told me don't ever put my finger on the phone and call her ever again."

"Wait, why? Why would she say that?"

Mama looked up at me. "Do it matter why? The fact remains that she's out of our lives. I just thought you should know."

And that was all she said about it. I never talked to Mother Rita on the phone, but I should have called her right then and there. I just kept thinking about the word Mama chose.

Our lives?

"LET'S STOP BY the drugstore first and get my pills," Mother Rita says. "Then I need to pick up some church bulletins from the printer. You want to go to church with me on Sunday?"

Though Mama grew up in the church down here in North Carolina, we were never regular churchgoing types in D.C., choosing more of a Christmas–Easter–Mother's Day kind of schedule, and I was the same with Shawnie and Darius when we were together.

47

"My flight leaves Sunday morning," I say.

Mother Rita ignores me. "After we leave the pharmacy, we can stop by the library. I got a couple of books under the seat here I need to return."

"Yes, ma'am," I say, enjoying the certainty her instructions give me. "Which way?"

"Wait a minute. Slow down." She lowers her window. "Hey, Maddie Mae!"

A silver-haired woman waves from her doorstep before walking over to the van. Mother Rita introduces us.

"This is my granddaughter, Veronica, the one using your boots. She's here visiting me from D.C."

"How you doing, nice to meet you, yes yes yes."

Mother Rita spends a few more minutes bragging. *She sells real estate in Washington. Her daughter graduated high school last year. Her mama doesn't get here much, but now she here to see about me.* She brags about me as if our family is simply a little too busy to visit often. I wonder if Maddie Mae knows more than she lets on, but she just nods and smiles and lets Mother Rita weave her family story out of thin air.

And I mean *thin* air. I'm definitely not the granddaughter she's describing. My marriage failed. My career has stalled. And clearly I haven't done the best job as a parent. Coming to visit Mother Rita may be my last-ditch attempt to do something useful for a change. If I can get her and Mama to make up once and for all, then maybe I can live up to these high praises.

The two women carry on a conversation that goes on so long you wouldn't think they live just down the road from each other. Maddie Mae says she already picked up the church bulletins so there's no need. Mother Rita asks her if she needs anything from the drugstore. I wait patiently, wondering how my mama behaved in this environment when she was around her mother, this country woman so comfortable in her own skin. It's hard to imagine Mama on this isolated road chitchatting as if there aren't appointments to keep.

"Okay, on to the drugstore," Mother Rita says to me when she's finished gabbing.

Walking down the aisle toward the back of the store, Mother Rita shares that years ago there was a family-owned operation in town, run by a Black pharmacist who not only knew you by name but could be so helpful when you described your symptoms. Back then, she says, the pharmacist might even examine you. She complains that the young people who work the pharmacy these days look tired and overworked and don't recognize her at all.

"Most times they have their noses stuck so far in a computer screen, it's hard to get a question answered."

I don't understand Mother Rita's complaints. Wearing wire-rimmed frames and a white coat, the pharmacist seems perfectly nice and does, in fact, recognize Mother Rita. "Would you like to wait while I put this together for you, Mrs. Lovejoy?"

"How long do you think it'll take? Anybody ahead of me?"

"I can get it done in ten minutes or so."

"That'll be fine."

We walk around the store and she buys a few things—a pair of pantyhose, a dustpan, some lip balm. They announce over the intercom that her prescription is ready. I follow her to the counter to pick it up, and I catch sight of the medication label. *Lortab.*

I recognize the drug from when I had my wisdom teeth pulled

years before. I remember all the warnings about its potency and the potential for addiction.

Why on earth is my grandmother filling an opioid prescription?

AS SOON AS we walk in the library, I know it's a place Mother Rita frequents often. The staff calls out to her by name. Even a couple of the patrons recognize her. Either Mother Rita is a local celebrity or this town is suffocatingly small.

The library has been recently renovated, and the odor of fresh paint hangs in the air. Spider plants fill an atrium framed by skylights. It's a weekday morning, so the tables are mostly empty. A lady with a silver ponytail and too-heavily-blushed cheeks stands behind the desk organizing a rolling stand of books.

"Hi, Mrs. Lovejoy. Bryan said you'd be stopping by. I believe he went out to get himself some lunch."

"Oh, that's fine. Here are my books."

I place her bag on the counter. Two cookbooks—one for pies and the other for Indian cuisine.

"I'll just look around while I wait for him," she tells the librarian.

"How long have you been vegetarian?" I ask her as we wander over to the stacks.

"I cut out meat years ago," she says. "Started with meatless Mondays. I had to figure out how to eat without meat and two sides on plate. At first, everything seemed like a bunch of side dishes. But eventually, I just looked to my garden. You eat meat?"

"Yes, ma'am," I say, sounding sheepish. In fact, I eat all kinds of processed food that would probably horrify her.

"Don't feel bad. To each her own. I ain't an evangelist about it."

She's graceful, too.

"I used to come here and read the newspapers. They even had a subscription to the *New York Times*. Now they only carry the local paper in print. Everything else is on the computers. Can you believe that?"

"You read the *New York Times*?"

She raises her eyebrows at me as if I'm from another planet, then waves her hand as if to say *pshaw* and moves between two rows of books in the fiction section, her eyes scanning the spines. My phone buzzes and I look down.

Any news? Offers?

It's my client texting me. The woman texts all the time with the same question. *No, I'm not a miracle worker,* I want to say, but she won't listen. Her house has been on the market for weeks now. The lovely June weather in D.C. was prime house-buying season, but we didn't receive a single offer. By the time they agree to lower the price, we'll be chasing the market and it might be too late. I really need to get back and do more marketing. Just the thought drains me.

I ignore my phone and follow Mother Rita into the stacks.

"My mama thought the public library was one of the greatest things the government ever did. She was so happy when the public library opened its doors to Black people. I was thirteen years old at the time, and we marched right down there to get my library card. You know old Ben Franklin was the one came up with the idea, don't you?"

One of my earliest memories with my mama was her taking me to get my public library card at the Petworth Library. But I never knew she'd gotten her love of the library from her mother, who'd gotten it from her mother.

"What was your mother's name?"

"Her name was Lily. Named after my grandmother's favorite flower. Didn't your mother ever tell you any of this?"

"No, she didn't."

"Well, did you ask her?"

I don't respond. Mother Rita shakes her head, as if to say *what a shame.*

A tall man in khakis and a white-striped collared shirt, dressed more like he is about to go golfing rather than working at a library, approaches and hugs Mother Rita. His beard is closely shaven with speckles of silver, but he doesn't look much older than I am. "Mother Rita, sorry I stepped out for a minute to get lunch. How you doing today?"

"Early for lunch, young man," Mother Rita teases.

He eyes me curiously. "Have we met before?"

"This is my granddaughter, Veronica, from D.C. No, you haven't met her yet."

He sticks out his hand. "Bryan."

"Nikki."

We shake hands, and as he turns back to the books, Mother Rita asks, "Any new fiction out?"

"Yes, ma'am, we just got in a new shipment." He guides Mother Rita out into the common area, where the new releases shelf is located.

I watch him walk off with her, noting how tenderly he holds her elbow. Mother Rita has real community here. That makes me feel better about being a neglectful granddaughter, but it also makes me feel a little jealous.

I wonder if any of these people—the neighbor, the librarian— clearly closer to Mother Rita than any of her own family members, know why she is taking prescription narcotics. And if she does need help with something, why hasn't she asked one of them?

SEVEN

Luella

The year was 1873, but we was still celebrating freedom. Life had never seemed so full of promise. Even when I gazed off into the distance, into miles of woods, it didn't frighten me. Our people was used to uncertainty. High up in these mountains, away from the lash of the law, free to move about as we pleased, we took nothing for granted.

In the midst of them first few months, me and William took our courtship slow. He didn't rush me, and I sure appreciated that because I wasn't ready. The women in the church watched him when they thought I wasn't looking. I might have been pretty, but William with his long-legged gait wasn't nothing to ignore.

At times, I glimpsed something fierce in his eyes, but he held himself steady, never allowing nobody to see too much of his in-sides. I saw enough to know that he had known his daddy and his daddy's daddy and that knowledge made him proud. The Mont-gomery men came from a warrior tribe, and that's why they was so tall. Maybe it was the warrior in William that made every word believable as gospel.

One cold December morning, on a day the winds was sweeping across the mountain with a fierceness most of us had not felt before, William gathered the kingdom dwellers at the tree to make an announcement.

"It's time we name our kingdom!" he shouted over the wind. "I say we call this place Happy Land. If this ain't the land of happy people, then where is it? Why not create our heaven right here on earth? Why not ask God to open the pearly gates right here on this mountain and deliver us?"

The man's ideas knew no limits. I had never heard a more perfect name.

"I lift mine eyes to the hills, said the Lord! Aren't these them very hills? What are we waiting on? People, our kingdom is now!" William's way of using language to help us create our new world was as powerful as any preacher's.

"Hallelujah! Hallelujah!" someone called out.

One by one, we began to lift our hands to the sky. A voice rose up in song, and though some of the words was lost to the wind, we swayed to the melody. Our Happy Land. Our paradise. It was as if my feet lifted off the ground. We was finally free—spirit free, body free. In that moment, we became something new yet again. How many times could we be birthed?

And then the men began to chant. *King William! King William!* And the women joined them. *King William!* while others called out *Mansa!*

I looked over at my papa, saw that his eyes was closed, and remembered how they'd tried to break him more than once. But here he was, standing alongside his people as we claimed our place on this rock, claimed our king and our kingdom.

It was a while before we left the tree that day. Nothing could move us, not the wind, not the cold. Even as we began to walk away, the new name of the kingdom still danced on our lips amid shouts of praise for our new king.

As I turned to follow Papa back to the cabin we shared, I saw William striding over to me, long legs making quick work of the distance.

"Marry me," he said in my ear, drawing close. "Be my queen."

"Queen?" I turned to face him, scarce believing what I'd just heard. The question seemed to drop from the sky. We wasn't even close to that yet. We had hardly done more than take a few walks together after Sunday services.

My hands was in my dress pockets, but he took one out and placed it on his chest inside his shirt.

"I know it sound quick. We ain't courted much. But I want to get to know you the right way, in God's eyes."

"Marry you?" I didn't know what else to say. Sometimes I couldn't believe I wasn't in South Carolina no more. Seemed like everything had changed overnight. We hadn't even been on this mountain but four months and here was this tree of a man asking for my hand.

"Luella Bobo, I want to be your husband. See after you. Be somebody you can lean on."

I sucked in the sharp air. "You talked to my papa?"

"Sure did. And he gave his blessing."

"Well, then," I said, too cold to spend a lot of time talking about it but wanting the moment to linger. "In that case, William Montgomery, yes, I will be your wife."

He lifted me up and twirled me twice. When he set me down I eyed him curiously. Now that he was out in the wilderness without all them white men breathing down his neck, he was gathering into new fullness as a man. People admired William, and so did I.

This must be how love feels, I told myself. *Comfortable. Respectful.*

He rushed off to begin his day's work. I glanced around to see if anyone had seen what just happened, but nobody was looking. Maybe this is what he had meant about claiming our kingdom right here on earth. Making our own choices, ruling our own lives.

Yes, it would be an honor to call King William my husband. I ran off to find Jola.

WE PLANNED FOR a springtime wedding, and it would come along at just the right time. The people welcomed the chance for a celebration. William asked his brother to help prepare for it. One day, when I arrived back at my cabin, the younger brother was waiting on the porch, having brought over a suit of clothes I could mend for William to wear on our wedding day. It was a decent cloth, and I knew William would look fine in it. I still hated sewing, but I would do this for my groom.

Robert's strong white teeth lit up his face, like rays of sunlight shooting out of his mouth. Unlike his older brother, who was quieter, with a serious face that didn't show much expression, Robert never seemed to stop talking. The man made me want to plug my ears with cotton.

"You and William about the same size. Can you try these pants on so I can see what need to be done?"

"Well you best turn around 'fore I start to think you being fresh with me," Robert declared.

57

I flushed with embarrassment as I turned. He should have just gone in another room. The man was plain rude.

He called out when he was ready, and as he held out his arms I slipped the jacket onto his shoulders, trying not to let my hands shake.

I pinched at the waist and ran my fingers under his arms. His body was warm to the touch though it was cold enough to freeze the tail off a horse outside. I stayed in back of him because I didn't want to look in his face too long, not wanting to get lost in them teeth.

"You seen Jola around?" I asked, to break the silence.

"Who?"

"She came here with us. Always wear that blue ribbon round her neck." Jola had scavenged her old mistress's room after she died. That ribbon had been with her ever since, and it was the one bit of fancy she allowed herself.

"I seen her around. She a friend of yours?"

"Since we was babies. Her mama knew mines."

"That right?"

I would need to take the coat in quite a bit for William. These Montgomery men didn't carry no extra on their bodies.

"Let your arms down." I squatted to check the hem of the pants. They was long enough, the two brothers built like rods.

He cocked his head back. "You get everything you need?"

I looked down. "I believe so."

He slipped the jacket off, and I held out an arm for him to pass it to me.

"I ain't said this to you yet, but I'm happy my brother found a woman he love. Seem like you a good woman."

I wasn't a good woman. I had just been rubbing my hands all

over the brother of the man I planned to marry. I wanted to ask what he meant by *seem like*.

"I wish I had found a woman like you." He laughed as if he was just joking.

"You ought to meet Jola." I stared at the floor, knowing good and well Jola wasn't interested in him.

"You have a pleasant day, Lu."

I followed him outside to the porch.

"It's Luella!" I yelled after him.

He turned briefly to flash teeth at me and I shook my head again, as if to refuse whatever bedevilment he was offering up.

FINALLY, IN MARCH, just as the ground began to thaw and the plantings started to bud, me and William married right there under God's sun. Papa performed the rites. Jola stood beside me wearing her blue ribbon. The sky was filled with noise—as if the birds had returned early just for the occasion.

William looked splendid in his jacket and pants. They made a sash of cloth for him to wear across his chest, sewed images of birds on the front with thread. When they brought the sash and crown to him for his approval, he praised them long and hard. William was quick to praise when kingdomfolk worked to please him. And they loved him for that.

William asked the women to make me a crown. So they gathered twigs and feathers and hung flowers to dry. They bound it all together with scraps of dyed cloth. I had to admit it was beautiful, though I felt it would be foolish to wear every day. Because I always wore my hair pinned up, Jola convinced me to wear it down, and it hung in a bush of curls around my shoulders. My dress was edged with lace, buttons running down the back. Widow Davis had gifted me the lace, and I'd been so overcome with emotion that my hands had shaken as I cut it.

Papa had taught me that choosing a husband was as much about survival as it was love. As I stood beside my groom underneath that oak, I knew that with him by my side, I would survive. William was a good man who possessed the kind of strength to see us through.

After Papa pronounced us husband and wife, William brought me to him tenderly and kissed me. It was our first kiss, and he acted like he didn't want to let me go. I was hesitant, shy. We turned to the gathered crowd as they erupted in a chorus of cheers.

One of the men started to scratch a fiddle, and music rang out in the air. I raised my skirt so it wouldn't touch the ground. William spun me around, the grin on his face wider than I'd ever seen it.

The scent of roasting hog wafted in the air. After the sun set, somebody lit a few torches and we carried on. Even Papa pulled up his pants legs, surprising us all with his quick dancing feet. We wasn't just celebrating a wedding, a legal union between husband and wife, we was celebrating the kingdom and the arrival of spring.

Each wave of an arm was a limb that belonged to you. Each step of a foot came from your own leg. We might have still been in the white man's country, but we was far, far away from his reach on that old mountain we called home.

Or so we believed.

QUEEN LUELLA.

I was still adjusting to my new role, still awkwardly talking to the other women as if nothing had shifted between us. I wore the same clothes as them, spoke to folks same as I always had. But they didn't stop to tarry with me much no more, keeping on about their business when they saw me. I couldn't decide if I liked this way of being treated, though William seemed to settle into it right away.

When the Widow Davis was told we was fashioning a kingdom led by a queen and king, they say she laughed but then sent down one of her dead husband's frock coats. William delighted in the gold buttons so much that he wore that wool coat even when the weather was too hot.

On Sundays, our day of rest, he walked around in his coat. It was not uncommon to hear a loud cheer from some corner— *Mansa!* Some of us had heard parents and grandparents tell stories of a king in England and his attempt to rule over here in America. Others, like William and his brother, spoke of a different kind of royalty, kingdoms in Africa.

Our memories was just dim enough that we knew we had to make our own traditions while trying at the same time to hold on to something. Our ceremonies wasn't from there, but they wasn't from here neither. We was all reaching for roots, holding on to some of the things we knew had marked us from the beginning— honoring our ancestors, paying respect to the land and the natural order, slapping a drum in tribute.

We had not played a drumhead at Lily of the Valley, and I wasn't sure who brought it with them to the hills. But once somebody started to play, it was as if we had known it all along. Our bodies responded to the drum as if spirits possessed. It became the call to eat, the call to warn, the call to celebrate.

How it was that African people came to these shores and created something new is not a riddle I can explain. But what I can

tell you is that we tried to create something in that place—
something we could call our own. Calling something your own is
a powerful prayer and there was God in it.

In his quest to shape our kingdom, William said that certain
things needed to set me and him apart from everybody else if we
was going to be respected. One thing he demanded was that we
didn't socialize after the evening meal. While others sat outside telling stories, me and William said our goodnights. What's more, we
had a larger house than most. Everybody said they was preparing us
for when the babies came by putting us in what they called a palace.

One night, a few weeks after our wedding, as we was preparing for bed, I could no longer bite my tongue. "William, I feel ri-
diculous wearing this crown. I don't need to wear it all the time."
No sooner than the words was out of my mouth, he struck me
across my face.

"You the queen, Luella. Start acting like it."

I covered my cheek with one hand, stunned and disbelieving.
I had never been struck before, not even during slavery. Papa had
always protected me from the worst in men.

"They don't remember no time of African kings," he said. "We
got to remind them of our strength."

I wanted to ask him if being a king meant fighting his woman
and where had he learned such a thing. But I tried to focus on his
words and not my stinging cheek.

We got to remind them of our strength.

I was pretty sure I understood what he meant. I just didn't
understand why he had to hit me to say it. I was not in disagree-
ment with him, but I remained silent.

EIGHT

Two years after I married William, I still wasn't pregnant. We didn't talk about it, but the disappointment sat between us like a log. As the women around me swelled with babies, shouting joy for children born into freedom, I said nightly prayers for one of my own. Every time a baby was born, they beat the drum. Two short rhythms followed by a shout followed by two short rhythms followed by another shout between wail and holler. If the baby was born in the middle of the night, a lone voice rung out to share the news.

My husband did everything to be gentle with me in them first two years, putting his apology for that fit of anger into deeds. Bringing me flowers because he knew I loved them. Washing my hair in the stream. Rubbing my back at night. He hadn't put his hands on me since that first time, but I carried the hurt on my back and it weighed me down like a rock. A part of me believed I couldn't grow a baby in my stomach unless I unloaded the ugly, but I never told a soul.

By and by, I forgave him.

In them days, when you was a woman without child, you had

no choice but to make yourself useful. Some of the people argued that the king and queen shouldn't work at all, that we should hold a place of honor. I didn't know what they expected us to do. Sit around and nap all day? That was not something we had ever known. In all of my days, I have to say, I have never met a lazy colored person. It was not something allowed of us. As soon as we could stand, we was required to meet the sun with a task. Of course, some of us hated the conditions more than others. Perhaps the ones who hated slavery the most, hated it with every inch of their bodies, was the ones called lazy.

Some of the work available to women in the kingdom included washing and mending, cooking, tending crops, canning for winter. As queen, I was given my choice of jobs. I would do most anything except mend and sew. I hated the needle.

I yearned for my own heralded announcement of a baby, but when that didn't come for me and William, I got to thinking about the children we already had in the kingdom, young ones who was working and helping out. I wanted them to learn their letters. I'd been able to learn mine, and I knew the magic in it. I suggested to William that we start a school, and he agreed. He wanted me to work on it so that by the time our children came, the school would be up and running.

First, I needed to get spellers. I asked the Widow Davis for help but she suggested I ask around about some free ones. When I asked Mr. Frank, the owner of the town store, he mentioned a school for white children on the outskirts of town. The walk to get to the school was long, but of course I didn't know that before I set out. The store owner hadn't shared the distance when he offered scant directions.

By the time I arrived, the back of my dress was soaked with sweat and my hair had come undone. I waited in the yard for school to finish, sipping water from my can. Outside the kingdom, I was no longer the queen. I was merely Luella.

The children poured out the door, and when one of them spied me, he called for the teacher. A woman wearing a blue dress emerged. "Excuse me, Miss," I began, hoping I was addressing her in the proper respectful tone. "I live in a colored community up in the mountains, and we would like to start a school."

"A colored community?" She glanced at my disheveled state. I could use a seat but I dared not ask.

"Yes, Miss." I tried to talk fancy, like my papa did when he was preaching. The trick was to talk a little faster.

"I was wondering if you got some old spellers or slates you don't use no more. Whatever you got will suit us just fine."

She paused. "I'm sorry, we use everything we've got. And we use the old spellers all over again with the younger children until we can afford new ones. We don't have much to spare."

"I understand. Just thought I'd ask. Thank you, Miss, for your time," I said, still talking faster than usual. I turned to walk away, my mind already running through other folks I might ask. Perhaps one of the travelers who came up the turnpike. Or one of the white churches. I didn't want to ask the treasury. There was still too many things for us to purchase with the little we did have. I tried to think of what I could trade.

"Excuse me?" she called out to me. "You never told me your name?"

"Luella."

"I'm Miss Ophelia. How about if I gave you one speller? I know it's not enough, but perhaps you could use it as a guide in your teaching."

One? There was already a dozen children in the kingdom, but I nodded before she could change her mind. "Yes, Miss. I would appreciate you."

"Give me a moment." She nodded to the boy to return inside and retrieve the book.

Perhaps the children could use it one at a time. I would figure out a way. One was better than none.

"God bless you, Miss."

She smiled at me. "God bless you, Luella."

SEEMED LIKE EVERY time I turned around Reverend Couch was bringing new arrivals. And the way their eyes lit up when they saw our settlement! Folks seemed so eager to join us, they got to work the same day they arrived.

Before long, we had nearly thirty children eager to learn to read and figure. One speller wasn't enough, but it would have to do. We didn't have a house so we decided we would hold class outside when the weather allowed, and when it didn't, there would be no school.

I had been leading the class, but we needed a proper teacher. I asked Reverend Couch if he would help find one on his next trip. We needed slates, too. If a teacher brought supplies, that would be even better. That was the best part about being queen. I could ask for things and everybody did their best to help.

What I didn't realize was that once folk got wind of my school project, the grown-ups would want some learning, too. So I started

Sunday evening school for them. Now we really needed a teacher. I hoped Reverend Couch would find somebody suitable.

I didn't know what kinds of tales Reverend Couch told the people he met about the kingdom, but he never seemed to have trouble finding them. The man returned with not one teacher but two. Sisters. And they'd brought slates!

In order to please William, I wore my crown when I met with the new teachers on the porch of my cabin. The sisters had similar names—Edwina and Eddy—but they would both be called Miss Jordan. I shared with them my vision for the school, how the children would study in the morning, leaving afternoons for chores; how eager adults would sit for class on Sunday afternoons.

"Say no more, Queen Luella," said the younger one. "What you have made here—this kingdom—is something special. We are ready to contribute our part."

"I can help walk the children up the hill," I said.

"That won't be necessary," replied the older one.

But I disregarded her and helped anyway during the first weeks. The younger sister was right. We was a special kind of community that worked together. That's just what we did in the kingdom.

ONE NIGHT, JUST after we'd finished our dinner, I decided to ask William about building a schoolhouse. He always pulled his suspenders down before he ate, and now they hung around his pants legs. We was so used to the food we'd eaten back in South Carolina that William demanded a lot from the women cooks in the kingdom. A group of women was in charge of the meals, and I daresay they was some of the best cooks I'd ever known. I often told them that South Carolina had lost its best cooks to North Carolina.

William was good and full, so I figured it was the right time to ask.

"Our little community growing. It's almost thirty children here. I think we need a proper schoolhouse." I picked up his plate.

William was quiet for a moment, as was his way. He leaned back in the chair and picked his teeth.

Many kingdomfolk would have liked to have private time to speak with my husband. William was known to give wise and generous counsel, but he was a man of little patience for idle chatter. Though he had been named king, he never ceased working. He still spent his days chopping wood, tending crops, and doing the same amount of work expected of all the men. At night he liked to sit quietly with me. I was always grateful for this alone time with him. Not every man would take this kind of time with his woman.

I went out to the porch to stack our plates so they could be picked up. When I returned, he was still sitting in the same position. "And the grown folk want some schooling, too."

He touched his beard. He had been growing it long ever since he became king. I thought it suited him even though I didn't like the feel of it against my face. There was crumbs in it from his dinner, and I resisted the urge to pick them out.

"Ain't y'all get the slates?"

"Yes, and I'm grateful for that."

"Ain't we got two teachers now?"

"Well, yes . . ."

"And the women already got a cookhouse. Now you talking about building a schoolhouse? We still figuring out how to feed everybody and get all our supplies. Everything cost money. Working for the Widow ain't enough. We trying to buy land, Luella."

"William," I interrupted, "you'd better put on extra bed-clothes. It's going to get chilly tonight."

While he got ready, I straightened the covers on our bed. William had built the bed himself, and it was a fine piece of work-manship. Timber in the area was quality, and he was a skilled furniture maker. The bed barely creaked when we lay in it.

I hung a pair of his pants and a shirt across the back of a chair for the next day. He liked for his clothes to be close by when he dressed in the morning because he often left the cabin before day-break.

I handed him a damp piece of cloth to wipe his hands and beard. Then I got myself ready. I figured it would be best to talk to him while we was lying next to each other. I blew out the wick, and we climbed in bed. He put an arm around me and I moved close to him.

"I know things cost money. Seed. Lamp oil. Flour and salt. And we can't depend on the Widow forever. The kingdom is grow-ing. But if the children—"

"None of that concern you. You supposed to—"

"The women can do it."

He turned to me sharply, and I saw something light his eyes even in the darkness. "Women can do what?"

"Build the schoolhouse. Why not? Y'all cut the trees and we do the rest."

I didn't know if we'd be able to lift the logs high enough for a house but maybe if enough of us tried together we could do it. Back in slavery times, women had done the work of men plenty times.

In the sliver of moonlight I could see William reach for the cover and pull it up to his neck, as if he was about to go to sleep without giving me an answer.

"William?"

His voice rang out, a hiss of air between his teeth. "You can't even bear me a child! You so busy trying to be a man that you ain't even half a woman!"

I turned from him and faced the wall. I had done everything to get pregnant, laying with William every chance I got even though the act left me feeling dry and empty. A tear slipped down my cheek.

He kissed me on my neck, as if in apology, holding me for a moment before letting go.

I thought of my papa's cabin, the warmth of the fire he made on cold nights. I would take off this crown and go back to my papa if William spoke to me that way ever again.

I curled my knees to my chest, waiting for my heart to slow and my lip to stop shaking.

ONE WEEK LATER, William woke up in his usual way, while it was still dark, but this time he woke me out of my slumber. One of the cooks usually left his morning meal on the porch, and since I didn't have to rouse to see him off, I stirred at the urgency of his voice.

"Luella, I got something to tell you."

I sat up and wiped the sleep out of my eyes. "What is it?"

"I'm going to work in the mines with one of the men today."

"The mines? Why you doing that? Ain't that dangerous work?"

"They say the money good, and we need it in the treasury."

I drew the cover over my legs. The mornings was chilly on the mountain. "I don't understand. We got plenty of men working out there. It's—"

"Luella, are you going walk me to the door or not?"

I slid to the side of the bed and stood on the cold floor. It didn't make sense to me that he wanted me to get up, but I did. He put his arms around my neck and whispered in my ear that he would be back.

I nodded and watched as he walked off with Hal Whitmire. William was acting strange, but I was so sleepy that I went back to bed without thinking too much on it.

It never crossed my mind that my husband wouldn't return that night or the night after or the night after.

NINE

Nikki

Mother Rita wakes up at sunrise to work in her garden. From the window, I can see her head bobbing up and down behind the garden fence. I tiptoe around the kitchen looking in cabinets, but I don't find any of her medicines. My mama keeps her medicine in the kitchen cabinet, but Mother Rita must keep hers in the bathroom inside her bedroom. I dare not enter her bedroom without permission, so I abandon the search. Maybe she's just taking the pain medicine for general aches. With all that stooping and working in the garden, surely she hurts.

I stuff my feet in the borrowed boots and leave out the back door. I want to see that graveyard again. I didn't get an accurate count of the stones, so I'm curious how many people are out there. We'd driven past Mother Rita's church, and I glimpsed a small cemetery in the back of it. Why hadn't our people been buried in a church cemetery? Wasn't that our family church? I'm ashamed of my ignorance.

Even through the boots, I can feel the morning dampness in my feet. Somewhere nearby, a woodpecker drums incessantly and I wish for Mama's binoculars. Once I arrive at the area of stones, I kneel and examine them closely. The rocks are smooth, as if they came from water. Without names, I don't know who I'm looking at, but I'm touched by a sense of holiness. This is sacred ground for my family. I graze the tips of the grass with my palm as I wonder about their stories. Who were my people, and what had they sought on this mountain?

I've never done any kind of family research, never had enough of a family to even know where to start, but now I'm beginning to realize, since arriving here, how much this missing hole goes beyond a decade-long spat.

I have so many unanswered questions. I sit on the ground, my bottom tight against its hard smoothness, and rub my face with the palms of my hands. Mother Rita is infuriating, but she's my grandmother, my flesh and blood. I stare down at my phone, feeling an urge to call Mama, but I don't have enough reception bars. I don't know what to make of this trip, this unfamiliar grandmother, this remote spot in the mountains where cell phones are not welcome.

Mama doesn't even know I'm here. Once she finds out she'll probably think I'm picking sides, as if that isn't the exact thing she has asked me to do all these years.

I stand and walk around so I can count the stones. It appears to be at least thirty graves. Husbands, wives, children, brothers, sisters. The old, the young. Natural causes, sickness, accidental death. I know none of the details; all I know is that these are my people. I stop at my grandfather's grave. Everybody buried on this mountain deserves the same respect, to have their names and years etched in stone same as his.

The ground isn't cleared, but it's covered in a hard dirt that makes it easier to walk through the brush. As I'm walking, the unmistakable *tik-tik* of a kingfisher draws my attention, and I catch sight of it just as it lands on a nearby branch. I track it from tree to tree with my eyes until it disappears.

I wouldn't call myself a birder, but as Mama likes to say, just noticing them is a start. I've never spent time in western North Carolina, but I've wandered the areas around D.C. looking for places to take a walk and watch birds. Mother Rita might think I'm all cityfied, but I'm not a complete stranger to the outdoors. I could spend hours out here.

The trees clear into a grassy flatness, and I continue walking, listening for birdcalls. My cell phone signal still isn't working, but I take pictures. I glance at my watch and realize I've been away from the house for over an hour. I don't want Mother Rita to worry, so I turn around and begin to walk back the way I came. She'll be finished in the garden soon. Maybe I can scramble up breakfast.

I look for the place in the trees where I exited and remember a pair of pines that stood together. I shade my eyes and scan the tree line. It takes only a minute or two for me to realize I'm lost. I could guess and just make my way and hopefully come out upon the house. Or I could continue walking until I arrive at a neighbor's house. I haven't seen a neighbor this far back on the land, but there has to be somebody.

I scan the ground, looking for signs of rocks that would mark the edges of the graveyard. A hawk swoops overhead, the legs of a small prey dangling from its beak. I stop to watch, unable to resist, but as soon as I do the hawk disappears into the treetops. I keep walking, glancing at my phone occasionally, hoping to catch a signal, and starting to get a little worried.

In the distance I hear the motor of a vehicle. I can't see it, but the muffled sound grows louder. It has to be some kind of all-terrain vehicle, because there's no road back here. I wait, hoping it'll be someone who knows my grandmother and the direction of her house. In these hills, everybody seems to know everybody. And we do have a private drive named after our family.

I wait until the ATV comes into sight and wave the driver down. As it draws close, a pale-skinned man wearing sunglasses raises a hand to his hat. All I have to do is ask about Lovejoy Lane, I tell myself, feeling unusually nervous. Surely this local person will be helpful.

"Good morning," I call out.

"Morning." He tips his hat, and I guess that he's slightly younger than I am. "You alright?"

"Fine, just a little lost," I say. "I'm visiting my grandmother and I cut through the trees. Now I can't find my way back."

He nods.

"I was out here looking at birds." I don't want to mention the graveyard.

"It's not like you're out here spying on the neighbors or anything, right?"

I give him a look, trying to determine if he's joking or being sarcastic. He has laugh lines around his eyes, and his shirt is tucked into freshly washed jeans. Only his boots are scuffed. Even his straw hat looks as if he carefully hangs it after he removes it. "If you consider birds your neighbors, then I'm guilty as charged," I try to joke in return, but it falls flat. "You live around here?"

"My house is a couple of miles that-a-way." He tilts his head. He hasn't offered to show me the way home, but I also haven't asked. I've already decided I'm going to hop into his vehicle to get a ride if he'll allow it.

75

"My grandmother's Lovejoy. Rita Lovejoy. Do you know—"

"Oh yeah, I know Mrs. Lovejoy," he says. "At least, I don't know her well, but our families have known each other for decades. You're her granddaughter?"

"Decades?" I repeat as I nod. Now I'm wondering what he's doing out here. I have an awful thought. What if his family enslaved ours? But I brush it off. This is the twenty-first century, I tell myself. All of that is long ago. The man is just a neighbor.

"You're here to help her pack up?" he asks.

"Pack up?"

"Never mind." He points to the seat beside him. "Hop in. I'll take you home."

I walk to the vehicle and swing a leg over the outside rail. It's like a golf cart, but louder and with bigger tires. Before I can say thank you, he takes off. He doesn't go very fast, but the ground is uneven and the vehicle bounces in the ruts. At some point, I lose my ponytail holder and my braids fly in my face. I can barely get my bearings as we take the long route to her house, passing through areas smooth enough to traverse. Finally, we come around to the grassy area behind Mother Rita's house, right next to her garden.

I climb off, trying not to stumble as I do. It's my first time riding in one of these and I'm a little dizzy, though I try to play it cool.

"Thank you."

"Sorry for the bumpy ride," he says.

"I'm sorry I didn't get your name."

"Al."

"I'm Nikki."

He takes off with a quick wave, and I watch as he grows smaller. I enter the house through the back door and pour a cup of coffee.

"So I see you met Fred Thomas's boy."

I jump. "You scared me. I didn't realize you were standing there. Yes, he gave me a ride back. I woke up this morning to go walk down to the graveyard, but then I . . ."—I point to the window, faintly realizing I was dumb enough to get lost in her backyard—"was looking at birds."

She places her empty mug in the sink. "He say anything to you?"

"Well," I stammer, unsure why this is all so awkward. "He said something about his family knowing you for decades."

She grunts.

"Are the Thomas family friends of yours?"

"If you call a snake a friend, I guess they are," she says.

She stuffs her hat on her head and threads her fingers into her gardening gloves. I can tell she's upset, so I quiet. The flash in her eyes is so dark that I believe I'm getting a glimpse of the woman who told Mama never to call her again in life. I wonder if the drugs make her moody. She must be in some kind of pain to be taking Lortab. "Breakfast is on the stove," she mutters before pushing the back door open and letting it slam behind her.

I take my coffee to the sunroom and sit in front of the window, appetite gone. Mother Rita exhausts me with her hot-and-cold mood swings. I look at the clock and pull my phone out of my pocket. All of my reception bars are back. I scroll through my Favorite contacts and eye Mama's name.

Then I remember what Al asked me, about helping my grandmother pack. What did he mean? Why would she be packing?

She's cantankerous, more than a little crazy, but she's intriguing. And I want to know more.

TEN

Just a couple of blocks from Main Street sits the Henderson County Public Library. The parking lot is full for a Tuesday afternoon. Sunlight streams through the skylights in the main reading room. I enter the glass doors and stand for a moment. It's intimidating to come here without Mother Rita and her strong, purposeful stride toward the fiction section. To my left is the audiovisual area, and to my right is a book display titled "Summer Reading Picks." I tell the librarian at the Research Assistance desk that I'm looking up local family history, and she directs me to the back. I walk between rows of book stacks and the wall, pausing for a minute to admire the local art on display. They're mostly landscapes, which makes sense—it's such a pretty setting to capture on canvas.

The room is named after Louise Howe Bailey. Four tables run down its center, and computers line the walls. I sit at one of the screens and move the mouse. It asks for a login. I look through my purse to find the library card Mother Rita gave me. Once I put in the number, I open a browser and type: Kingdom Happy Land Henderson County.

A few results pop up. Brief website posts. A few local newspaper articles. All of them appear to reference a person named Sadie Smathers Patton who wrote an account of the kingdom published in 1957, but when I try to search for it online, I can't find the full text.

I open another tab and type in my grandmother's name: Rita Lovejoy. Nothing. I should have known. Anybody without a computer certainly wouldn't have an Internet presence.

"Good morning."

I turn around. Mother Rita's librarian friend is looking over my shoulder at my screen. I understand there's no privacy in a public computer space, but I'm annoyed that he snuck up on me.

"Sorry, I was, um, looking for something Mother Rita mentioned." I find myself explaining my presence instead of saying hello. There's no surreptitious way to close my browser with him hovering over me, so I don't even try.

"Oh, you thought I was looking at your screen, didn't you?" He laughs. It's a nice sound. Warm and easy. "I was trying to check and see if you needed any help with anything. I saw you come in, but I was working with somebody."

"Good morning. I guess I should've started with that."

He sits down in the chair beside me. "I found a book for you, actually." He jumps back up. "Let me go get it."

He leaves and returns after a few minutes, carrying a small paperback. "It's a local guide to flowers. I figure you might want to learn something about your grandmother's garden."

"Actually, I downloaded an app on my phone."

"Oh," he says, looking disappointed.

"But thank you. I'll take a peek. It looks interesting." I tap the cover to reassure him.

"I could get you a book on birds. Mrs. Lovejoy told me your mother is a bird-watcher. Maybe you like them, too?"

I stop breathing for a moment. Mother Rita has been talking about Mama's bird obsession. That's a good sign. All those questions about Mama and now this confirms it. She misses her daughter. Perhaps that means there's hope for a reconciliation.

Bryan carries on as if he hasn't noticed my thoughts slipping away. "I like taking walks, too. But sometimes I forget to look up. Y'all birders remind me of that."

I place the guide on the table beside me. "Sometimes I forget to look down. I'm so busy looking for the birds up in the trees that sometimes they're right in front of me, watching me instead of me watching them. You know, some of them are ground nesters."

"Or maybe they're just walking around minding their own business. Like I should be doing right now."

"No, don't worry, you're fine," I say.

"I'm sorry for walking up on you like that."

I touch him on the arm. "You're fine."

He appears to relax, smiles at me. "So you're a birder, huh?"

"Well, I don't carry binoculars or anything."

"What's your favorite?" he asks.

"Now, that's an impossible question," I say. "I've got a few."

"Okay, have you seen anything interesting around here yet?"

"I did see a pretty kingfisher out back of Mother Rita's property this morning."

"Nice. Out on that mountain, you're certain to see ones y'all don't get in the city."

"If you have a local bird guide, I'll be grateful." I don't want to tell him that I have an app on my phone for birds, too. Our eyes lock for a moment. I can see why Mother Rita likes him so much. He has a sincerity about him. When he looks at me, it's as if he really sees me. Maybe he's just one of those curious people. I peel my eyes away and turn back to the screen. "Hey, I do actually have a question. Do you know anything about this Sadie Smathers Patton? I'm reading about her and she—"

"So Mother Rita told you about the kingdom, I see."

"You know about it?"

"Of course. All the locals do."

"Is it—is it just a bunch of folktales? I mean, I know our family lived on that land, but a king and queen seems so . . . far-fetched."

He nods. "From what I can tell, it's all true. I know it sounds crazy, but think about it. There have been other Black intentional communities in this country."

Intentional communities. That's an interesting phrase. "Oh yeah? Like where?"

"In Mississippi there was a community known as Mound Bayou. At its height, there were about four thousand people living there. They had their own government and schools. And on the border of Kentucky and Tennessee there was the Coe Ridge Colony. It was established after the Civil War and lasted all the way up to the 1950s."

I study his face with a newfound respect. "I've never heard of any of this."

"Don't feel bad. There are a lot of people who've never heard of them. I'll try to find you some books. In the meantime, Sadie Patton's account is right here."

He plucks a pamphlet off the bookshelf next to us. All along, I'd been sitting right next to it. "You can't check it out of the library because it's considered reference material, but you can read it right here."

"Of course."

"It's a long story. Generations old, I'm afraid. How long you going to be in town?"

"I leave on Sunday."

"You should stick around. Ask Mother Rita some of these questions while you're able."

"While I'm able? Mother Rita may be seventy-eight, but from what I can tell, the woman's mind is sharp enough to cut cheese."

He nods slowly. "After you take a look at Patton's version, you might want to go through some of those old slave schedules. Work from there forward and maybe you can trace their path."

He pulls up a site and moves to stand as I squint at the screen. "Okay," I say, wishing he would stay with me and show me step-by-step.

"Hey, let me know if you need anything else. I'm here all day and happy to help you with anything at all, hear?"

I know he has to get back to work, but as he walks away I want to call him back and pretend I have another question. Clearly, this man is more than a librarian. Or maybe I don't know enough librarians.

I place Patton's pamphlet on the table beside me and open another browser tab. My fingers hover over the keyboard. I want to learn more about this Queen Luella and how she came to rule the kingdom, but the first thing I need to figure out is her story. Though I'm elated at the idea that my people owned land, I want to know why they came up that mountain in the first place.

As I scroll through the library databases, the stops and starts frustrate me. I pick up Sadie Patton's account and start reading until a story emerges. According to Patton's version, the group originated in Mississippi, and after Emancipation, with a dream of freedom spread out before them, they followed an itinerant preacher up the mountain to establish a community where they could rule themselves. She uses the phrase "One for All, All for One" as a slogan to represent their dream.

Patton says as the original kingdom settlers moved north, their numbers grew along the way. That's a long walk. Surely there are plenty of remote spots they could have stopped. But I'd walk to the ends of the earth to make a new life for me and Shawnie and that's no exaggeration.

Even so, I'm surprised Patton insists on Mississippi, because Mother Rita believes the original settlers came from South Carolina and suggested that's where I should start my research. So I look up the name Bobo in the Federal Slave Schedules. I've never looked at one of these, and deciphering the handwriting is next to impossible. None of the people are recorded by name, only by age, sex, and color. One column asks if the person is a "fugitive from the state." Even if the person ran off to claim their personhood, they are still listed as "property" in the census. The next column is more hopeful: "Number Manumitted." But I never see a single instance in the schedules where someone has been freed.

One asks if the person is "deaf & dumb, blind, insane, or idiotic." Every time I see a mark in this column, I wonder about the meaning. There are even a few children noted as such, as casually as if noting a crack in an egg. I feel a headache coming on. I'm just trying to find my great-great-great-grandmother, and I've got to wade through trauma. Maybe this is why a lot of Black people don't know our history. Just the search requires fortitude.

Something catches my eye. In the 1860 schedule, Elizabeth Bobo of Cross Anchor owned a thirty-four-year-old man and a ten-year-old girl. Neither person is named, but the age of the little girl sounds right. Could that be Luella and her father?

THAT NIGHT MOTHER Rita and I set up dinner in her back sunroom. A vinyl tablecloth with strawberries printed on it covers the table, and she has mixed up a fresh batch of lemonade. I've prepared a simple pasta, broccoli, and garlic bread. I'm not an extraordinary cook by any measure, though from Mother Rita's excitement, you would think the meal had been cooked by an executive chef.

"Bryan tells me you stopped by the library today."

I look up, startled again by how quickly news travels.

"You find anything?" she asks.

"I read the Patton pamphlet. I'm assuming you know about it?"

"Course I do."

"She says they came all the way from Mississippi. But for the life of me, I can't find any evidence of that."

"That's 'cause they didn't. The kingdomfolk were from South Carolina."

"So why would Patton say that?"

"Why do people write fiction? It feeds the imagination. Maybe she didn't want to say the real reason they came up here, how the Klan in South Carolina made their lives a living hell. I don't know.

Look, she was a 1950s white historian trying to document the kingdom. She did her best, but I'm sure she had her blind spots."

I pick up my phone, where I saved a few notes. "You mentioned that Luella's husband was a Montgomery. There was a Montgomery down in Spartanburg County who died in 1864. She left a will leaving her estate to her daughter. But I think somehow her brother claimed some of the people." Seeing those people listed alongside farm equipment, furniture, and animals was misery.

"So you're learning slavery was outlawed but people carried on."

"Bryan says that even though the Emancipation Proclamation was issued in 1863, South Carolina didn't recognize it until the end of the Civil War."

"Yes, that sounds about right." Her eyes glitter. She is listening carefully.

"So then I looked for her brother J. D. Montgomery's name in the 1850 and 1860 schedules. Between those two decades, he increased his holdings from eighteen to thirty-five. And among those listed are two boys, ages fifteen and eighteen. I think that's Robert and William."

"The brothers I told you about."

"Exactly."

"So now you've got to find Luella."

I rise and go to my room to retrieve the folder Bryan gave me, containing a few photocopies. I know Mother Rita is more interested in Luella than anything.

When I return, she has opened a bottle of wine.

"Are you supposed to be drinking?" I ask, thinking of her medication.

"Mind your business. Now, what you got there?"

I open the folder and slide it across the table to her. "I found Martin Bobo in a federal slave schedule for Cross Anchor, South Carolina."

"And a girl," she whispers, reading it. "My mama told me Luella's daddy was a preacher."

"Sometimes Luella's name is spelled differently, depending on the source."

"Those census takers didn't always ask how to spell a name, especially when it came to our people."

"It doesn't appear that the census takers went into the kingdom. So once they walked up that hill, I lost track of them."

"They probably didn't let government people on their land." She takes a final bite of pasta, cleaning her plate. "But you've got to figure out how Luella came to rule the kingdom. They say she ruled it above even the king."

"That might be impossible to know."

"You know what was impossible? Walking up that mountain and making a home. You know what else was impossible? Becoming a Black queen in the United States of America. Don't tell me about impossible."

"I'm doing the best I can, Mother Rita."

"Look, don't get me wrong. You're good at this. You should've gone to college."

Her words mollify me. "I must say there's something thrilling about every little discovery. It's like with each puzzle piece, I'm one step closer to putting my own bones together." I surprise myself with the metaphor.

"Bones, huh. That's a way to put it." She takes a long sip of her wine. I watch as she empties the glass and refills it, but I don't say anything.

"If Patton didn't get the Mississippi part of the story right, maybe her insistence about the king and queen is also made up. I mean, we don't really know for sure—"

Mother Rita brings my attention back to her with a firm grip on my forearm across the table. "Babygirl. You've got to believe. Otherwise, we're just over here kicking up dust."

"Believe in what exactly? Mother Rita, why is all this so important to do on this trip? I mean, why the urgency?" Mother Rita has me down here on a wild goose chase searching in the archives, claiming it will answer my questions about her and Mama. She's right about one thing: I don't know what to believe.

She must be able to tell she is losing me, because she lets go of my arm and places both elbows on the table. "Veronica, listen. What I've been trying to tell you is that they stole it."

"Stole what?"

"Our land. The land our ancestors owned, that Luella owned."

I put down my fork. "Wait a minute. What are you saying? Don't you still own this house and property? Didn't they pass it down in our family?"

My grandmother's eyes don't look like she's tipsy from the wine. They're clear as glass.

"No, I don't own it. That's what I'm trying to tell you!"

"Well, who took it? And when? Are you paying rent to somebody to live here?"

"No, I don't pay no rent," she snaps. "I haven't owned this land in twenty years, but it's still mine. *Ours*. You're a real estate agent and know about property. It's why I called you for help."

Now I'm really confused. "If you don't possess the deed to the land, Mother Rita, it no longer belongs to you."

She shakes her head. "It's our land, Veronica."

"Help me understand how you can believe that."

"I need you to help get the land back. Do you see now? It's what Luella wanted for us." She raises her glass and shouts, "Here's to taking back our land and our birthright!"

I almost choke on my food at her sudden outburst. This might be kingdomland, but it's also crazyland.

ELEVEN

In the middle of the night, Mother Rita wakes me up and tells me she isn't feeling well.

"Not feeling well how?" I say, barely awake but straining to focus.

"I called my doctor. He didn't answer."

I look at my watch. "It's four o'clock in the morning. You called his office?"

"No, girl. I called my doctor at home. Didn't you hear me? Ain't you listening?"

I swing my legs to the side of the bed. "Okay. We need to go to the emergency room. If he calls back on the way there, you can talk to him then."

I expect her to protest. Nobody likes going to the ER in the middle of the night. When she doesn't, I know it's serious. "I'll throw on some clothes and meet you in the front room."

She nods and moves slowly out of the room. As I pull on my jeans, I try to clear my brain fog. I take out my wallet and clip a long strap on it, turning it into a crossbody bag. Better to travel light in case things take a turn.

In the front room, Mother Rita sits in an armchair, already dressed in a pink velour tracksuit. A book peeks from the top of a brown canvas tote.

"You've got your insurance card and ID?" I ask.

"Child, sure. This ain't my first trip to the rodeo."

After we get in the car and buckle into our seats, I pick up my phone, ready to navigate. "Which hospital?"

She closes her eyes. "Turn left," she says.

I try not to let my old memories around Daddy's sudden illness crop up. Mother Rita appears healthy, but there is that mysterious pain med prescription. I should have just asked her about it.

There is still so much I want to know about her. I glance over, wanting to ask how she feels, but her eyes are still closed and I don't want to disturb her. At a stoplight, I take a longer look. Her expression is wrinkled and stressed.

"Left and then your first right."

I turn. The streets are empty, streetlights blinking red. Signs appear, indicating the direction of Pardee Hospital, so I won't need to wake her for the last few minutes of the drive. I have a brief moment of panic as I consider that I should've called an ambulance.

At Fleming Street and Bearcat, the road leads directly into the hospital entrance. I follow the signs to the emergency entrance and park in the visitors' parking deck, unsure if I should unload her at the door or if she can walk.

She opens her eyes and passes her tote to me. "That little nap did me some good. Can you take my bag?"

"Yes, of course. You want me to pull up to the door?"

"No, baby. I'm fine. Just come take my arm."

I quickly move around to her side of the car and take her arm in mine. She greets the attendant at the ER entrance by name, and when I looked at her quizzically, she explains, "Her mother is the county clerk." Once again, I am reminded of the circles of community here.

We sit beside one another in green vinyl chairs in the waiting room. There is a small room to the side containing a vending machine that hums loudly. I watch as a nurse calls someone into one of the three triage rooms.

Looking up at the television, Mother Rita says, "Don't worry too much. I'm just feeling a little sick to my stomach."

"Do you think it's that wine you drank?" I ask softly, worried that I should've stopped her.

"Hell no. Wine is good for you, comes from grapes."

I'm paralyzed with fear. I want Mother Rita to read more books, grow more flowers. I want her to see Shawnie again. I want her and Mama to reconcile. The strength of my hopes for her surprises me when all I've felt since I arrived is frustration.

"You think it's your medication?" I try to come in sideways.

"Could be." Typical Mother Rita, casting the conversation on her terms. It's just her way, I'm learning, so I strain to give her the benefit of the doubt. She probably doesn't feel well enough to talk about it.

On television there's a rerun of an entertainment show. Mother Rita only watches the news, so I doubt she recognizes any of the celebrities.

"Do you ever go to the movies?" I ask her, trying to keep her mind off her distress.

She shakes her head. "I'm not much of a moviegoing type."

For a while I was dating a neighbor who had a TV so large it overwhelmed his small living room. He was obsessed with Pablo Escobar movies until one time I reminded him that Colombia was more than a setting for drug cartels. The relationship ended soon after. Now my online dating profile is out of date, and I haven't gone out with anyone in almost two years. When Shawnie was in high school, I used her as an excuse. These days my romantic life is about as stale as my work life.

I wonder what other treasures lie within Mother Rita's mind. Though none of us has a degree, we're hardworking people who have made our way. Mama is a well-respected federal employee. I sell houses and support my daughter as a single mother. We have health insurance and retirement funds. Still, I can't help but imagine what we might have done with more education.

We wait for almost three hours. Bored, I begin to study the people in the waiting room. A woman in black-rimmed glasses with curly hair teased into a hive. A grandfatherly man in a security uniform, his shirt unbuttoned at the neck. I'd always thought of Hendersonville as some far-off place. Completely different from my life in D.C. These are the hills, after all. Appalachia. These people are supposed to talk different. Dress different. Act different. But they look like everybody else I've ever known. I'm not sure why that strikes me in this moment, but it does. We are all the same, I think.

"Mrs. Lovejoy? We're ready to take you back."

I stand with her, but Mother Rita touches my arm.

"I'll call for you if it's necessary. You go on home. Eat something and get a little sleep."

"But Mother—"

"Bryan lives close by. Between the both of you, I'll be fine."

I hesitate. Everybody knows you get better care in hospitals when you have family around. But Mother Rita's sharp eyes don't appear open to negotiation at this early morning hour, so I hold my tongue. I am tired. The vending machine potato chips float like air in my stomach.

"I need you rested, baby. I might be here a few more hours. Now, look"—she takes my hand in hers and squeezes it hard—"don't go doing nothing foolish like calling your mama. I'll be home before dinner."

I nod and blink. Then I watch helplessly as she follows the attendant down the hall.

AS EXHAUSTED AS I am, I can't go right to sleep when I get back to the house. The morning sun streams brightly through the windows, and my eyes are dry and itchy. I walk through the house, touching Mother Rita's things and feeling her absence. It's the first time I've been in the house without her either sitting somewhere reading or working out back in the garden. I walk down the hall to her bedroom. Usually, she keeps the door open when she isn't in there, but it's closed now. I guess she didn't feel like tidying up before leaving, and when I open the door, I see that I'm right. I've walked past the room countless times in the last few days, but I've never entered, out of respect. The four-poster bed is always perfectly made, a pink coverlet spread neatly, with pillows tucked at the head. She makes her bed the old-fashioned way—there are no lumbar or decorative pillows. The sight of the rumpled covers unsettles me.

I inhale my grandmother's scent. A light floral like rose water. The pink wall-to-wall carpet is clean, but it could stand to be

93

replaced. The bed is a dark wood, and I place a hand on one of the poles, my fingers slick against the furniture polish. A stack of books sits on the bureau. I scan the spines: two by Maya Angelou, one by Toni Morrison, and a fourth by someone named Randall Kenan. I pick up the book and a handsome, smiling Black man looks directly at me from the author photo. Beside the books, dried purple flowers shoot from a small vase. A mirror hangs above the dresser, which is adorned with crochet doilies and trays holding an array of lotions.

Her bathroom is tiny, as if it was originally a walk-in closet. A black-and-white tile walk-in shower and a pedestal sink. Matching pink towels. I pick up a jar on the shelf above the sink and open it. Some kind of essential oil. Bergamot? I quickly put it back, feeling a little guilty for having touched her things. I am just so curious about this woman.

I sit on Mother Rita's bed, the scent of her still in my nostrils. I think of calling to check on her, but it has barely been an hour since I left the hospital. I should probably call Mama, but considering Mother Rita's warning, I decide to wait until I know more. Fatigue weighs down my eyelids.

I wake to the sound of my cell phone ringing; 9:17 a.m. glows on my phone. "Hello? Hello?" I've fallen asleep in Mother Rita's room on top of her coverlet.

"Hey, did you get some sleep? I'm just calling to tell you they admitted me. But everything's fine. I'm just getting some fluids and then they'll let me come home. Don't you worry about me none."

"Did they say why you were feeling sick last night?"

"Well, we know why, baby. I got cancer."

"Mother Rita." I inhale sharply, suddenly wide awake as I sit up. "You have cancer? Where?"

Ever since Daddy died of cancer, this has been my worst nightmare for the people in my life. My eyes well with tears, and the effort to hold them back makes my whole face hurt. I shake my head a little and blink.

"It started in my lymph nodes," she says.

"Started?"

"Honey, I'm too old for chemo."

"What does the doctor say?"

"Too old!" she yells into the phone.

She has delivered this news the way she reveals everything. With brutal clarity. No wonder she has the Lortab prescription. I try not to let her hear me sniffle as I pull her pillow to my face, but all it does is fill my nose with her rose scent again. I've only been here three days, and I'm just getting to know her. When daddy got his cancer diagnosis, he was gone within a year. If Mother Rita's cancer has spread—

"Have they put a clock on it, Mother Rita?" I have been through this before. I know when death is knocking at the door. This must be the real reason she has asked me to come, why she showed me the family graveyard and told me to bury her there. This is why she wants to know if Mama is okay. All to settle her family accounts.

While she's still able. That's what Bryan said. He knows.

"They say months, but what do they know? They told me that at the first of the year and here it is July already."

"They told you this in January?" I'm panicked. Mother Rita doesn't look sick to me, but I don't know what she looked like before. She is literally dying, and I can't let that happen without all of us getting together.

"Get a hold of yourself, Nikki. I'm not planning to go anywhere anytime soon." This is the first time she has used my preferred name, and it slows my whirl of thoughts. "Now, you got to cut the flowers and take them to market this week. Maddie Mae'll help you. Her grandson usually set up the tent and table for me, so customers can buy straight out the buckets. All you got to do is wrap them. And check the mail for anything official-looking. Bring it to me when you bring my dinner."

"What? You want to sell flowers this week? And you want me to bring your dinner?"

"You don't expect me to eat this garbage they serve here, do you?"

"No, ma'am." I try to pull myself together. She demands no less. "Anything special you want to eat?"

"I'm not picky," she says in exactly the tone that says she is, in fact, picky. "Just whatever you feel like rustling up." That means something homemade, not fast food. She seemed to enjoy my food last time, but my skills in the kitchen are limited.

As if reading my mind, she says, "And I eat anything grow out of God's green earth. Anything."

"Yes, ma'am," I respond.

I NEED TO go to the supermarket and figure out dinner for Mother Rita, but I can't seem to will myself to move fast enough. Everything is in slow motion, including my body. I scoop coffee into the coffeemaker, and it feels like thirty minutes to make one cup. I sit at the kitchen table, pick up my phone, and scroll to Favorites. I've texted Shawnie a couple of times, but she hasn't responded. I decide to call. I need to hear her voice.

She picks up right away. "Hey."

"What you doing?"

"I'm at work."

Shawnie is working part-time at a bakery, but they give her less than twenty hours a week. She has been out of high school a year, and she really needs to figure things out. But I'm too tired to lecture her right now.

"How's work going?"

"It's fine. I can't talk, Mama. They don't like us on our phones. I just answered to see if everything is okay."

I want to say, no, it isn't. I want to tell her the news of her great-grandmother's illness, end the years of silence creating a thick cloud between the Lovejoy women. But I can only bring myself to say, "Everything's fine."

I have been a mother most of my adult life, and I never lie to my daughter. So I don't know why I don't tell her about Mother Rita's diagnosis. I tell myself that I don't want to panic her, but I know that isn't true. "You eating alright?"

"Yes, I'm eating. Now, did you solve all the mysteries of the family yet?"

If only she knew. Shawnie is curious about the family dynamics, but since it's all she's ever known, it doesn't seem to bother her as much. "I'm working on it." My voice cracks, but she doesn't seem to notice.

"Okay, I've got to go."

"Love you, Shawnie."

"Bye."

After she hangs up, I stare at the kitchen wall. My mouth opens, as if I'm about to say something, but nothing comes out. Talking through hurts was never easy for my mama, and I guess it isn't easy for me either. I need to call Mama, but I don't move.

TWELVE

Luella

At first, the men told me William was planning to stay the week in the rooming house for the mine workers. Then they told me he would stay the month. Soon it became apparent that my husband wasn't coming back no time soon. But I was still in denial. He was the king. Of course he would return.

I went to Robert, desperate for news. *Have you checked on your brother?* I wanted to know. Robert assured me he was fine, but when I asked about the date of William's return, he was silent. I tried to continue my work, act as if nothing was the matter. I had not given my husband children and he had left me. William Montgomery loved being king, but maybe he'd wanted to be a father even more. Maybe he'd taken another woman and was bringing her back to take my place. All kinds of thoughts rushed through my head.

One morning I rose and wiped the sleep out of my eyes. I would go see about William for myself. If he wanted to replace me, he would have to tell me to my face. The mines was far, so I tucked a coin Papa had given me on my wedding day inside my dress.

Walking down the hill to the gate, I heard footsteps behind me.

"Don't try and stop me," I said to whoever was following.

"I didn't come to stop you."

"I don't need you to walk with me. I know the way," I replied, recognizing Robert's voice.

"I ain't going with you," he said.

"So why you here, then?" I stopped and turned.

He approached me and took my hand in his. I snatched it back.

"I come to tell you the truth."

He was about to give me bad news, I could feel it. "Tell me. Is William . . . dead?"

He shook his head quickly, and I let out a whistle. I had been holding my breath and hadn't realized it.

"He got hurt in the mines, didn't he."

When he finally looked me in the eye, I broke off in a run.

"Stop, Lu! Wait!"

When I reached the gate, I slowed, my heart pounding. Robert easily caught up.

"Stop it. Let me go." Sweat dripped down the center of my back as he wrapped an arm around me.

"There was an accident. Something fell on his head—"

"What you mean an accident? When? How long y'all been hiding this from me? I got to go to him. He alive, right. He can just come back here and I'll help him."

"Lu, he blind. He can't see."

"You say he blind?" I tried to think. So he was still able to walk. He was just hurt and too shame to come back?

"He my brother, the closest person in the world to me, but I can't speak for him. I just know he don't want to come back right now. And he don't want you coming down there neither."

"But he can't see and he needs me. Who's helping him? How's he managing?"

He shook his head again, and by the look in his eye, I knew I couldn't go. William needed time. That's what Robert was trying to tell me.

I turned back up the hill. There was nothing more to say or do. If William didn't want me, then it didn't make sense for me to go after him. I would just have to wait.

THERE WAS TWO widows now. Me and Serepta Davis. Her husband had long ago died, but we still referred to her as the Widow. She seemed to like the title, though she had shed her mourning attire months after we arrived. She was a widow by death, but I was a widow by abandonment. When she heard news of William's departure, she was kind enough to send me a fresh loaf of bread. I could barely eat it.

No one spoke of what would happen next. I expected I would be asked to move out of the palace soon, so I packed my things. Papa had gotten used to having his own house, but he told me I was always welcome. The council was set to discuss naming a new king.

I worried what would happen to the kingdom. William had been the one to bring us here in the first place, to set the vision for us. Jola quietly mentioned I should run the kingdom as queen. She said the other women agreed. But women was not even allowed on the council, and it was impossible the men would ever consider such a thing. I'd watched William and how he had, with his soldier's posture and deep knowledge of numbers, inspired loyalty among the people. He had been an imperfect husband, but a fine leader.

I tried to get my mind off William by going over ideas for the kingdom in my head. Surely I knew how to get things done. I'd shown that when I started the school and brought in the teachers. William had pushed the men to work outside the kingdom. But I believed that unless we was creating our own work, we would be dependent on white men and their wages forever.

I took out William's ledger, which I knew showed the crops and land parcels he'd assigned each family, and asked Robert to come over and help me decipher it after he finished work for the day. He agreed.

"Let's sit out here on the porch while there's still light," I said. Robert pulled a chair next to mine, close enough that the scent of him reached my nostrils. A whiff of grass and earth.

"What you hoping to get out of this?" Robert asked.

"I want to figure out how we can work right here in the kingdom so everybody don't have to keep going down the hill to earn wages."

"Some of the land ain't good for growing. We need oil for lamps and grain for bread. Coffee and such. What ideas you got?"

"Can you help me figure out William's numbers? I thought maybe you knew how he wrote all this."

I passed him the book. After looking it over, he said William had been estimating how long it would take to save enough to buy land. Owning land meant more houses, more families, more crops. But the land was more than just houses. It was how we could build a life. Without it, we was rootless.

"That's all?"

"The land ain't no small thing. What else on your mind?" He sat back in the chair and looked at me. Robert wanted to hear what I had to say, and his belief gave me courage. He ran a long finger down the page as he read. His nails was short and clean, as if he'd never touched dirt.

"What if we made something and sold it. A lot of travelers go up and down that turnpike, and we been trading already. But what if we made something everybody needs. Something they would pay for."

He scratched the hairs on his chin. "Like what?"

"I-I don't know," I admitted. We had such limited tools. Even the blacksmiths who was hired out used the tools they was given.

"I hope you ain't talking about making hooch. The Widow already told us she won't allow nothing of the sort."

"No, not hooch, Robert!"

He laughed. "You never called me that before."

"What?"

"By my name."

"What did I call you?"

"Nothing, I guess."

I tried to ignore him. "There has got to be something we can make."

He looked down at the book. "Right now the men finding work outside the kingdom. The railroad. The inn. Hauling up and down the turnpike. You want to pull them off?"

"No." I shook my head. "At least, not yet. Maybe there's something the women can make."

"Like what, Lu?"

"I don't know. Soap or something. Everybody need soap. And I asked you not to call me Lu. Only my papa call me that."

"Okay, Queeeeen." He drew the word out, and a glint of mischief sparkled in his eyes.

"Any word from your brother?"

He cleared his throat several times, as if something lodged in it just as he was about to open his mouth and lie. I squinted at him. "Nothing since we talked," he managed to croak out between swallows.

"I'd like to send him word."

"I'm sure that can be arranged."

"Tell him I'm moving back in with Papa soon as the new king is chosen. He can find me there." Surely William would be back soon as he got over his shame. It had been months, but I was certain my husband would return before winter.

Robert didn't say nothing. He just watched me.

THE COUNCIL WAS scheduled to gather just after sundown. It was a Sunday evening, our day of rest, and some of the men was still at the schoolhouse receiving their lessons. The council would gather at the tree as they always did. They'd sit on seats carved out of stumps. They'd begin with a report on the community's news, moving on to address complaints, settle disputes. But on this particular night, they would also discuss a new king.

Just before sunset, Robert knocked on the door of my cabin. I opened the door right away; I'd already been expecting somebody would call on me to remind me it was my last night in the palace, either way the wind blew. I was all packed and ready to go.

"Can I have a word?" Robert asked, a dusty hat in his hands.

I invited him inside but left the door open. I didn't know why I did that, but I did.

"Have a seat," I said, motioning to the chair. He sat down as I busied myself straightening things. I had begun putting together

William's clothes to send by one of the mine workers, but I would leave William's royal coat and sash for the new king. Whoever took the throne would want them. I was also leaving behind my crown. I'd never liked wearing it, but I still felt a little melancholy about the way things had turned out. "I ain't told you this, but I'm grateful you delivered the news about your brother. I was eaten alive with worry."

"That wasn't easy news to give, and I know it wasn't easy to take," he said.

"I figure you asking the council for consideration tonight. That's why you here. To know if you got my backing."

"My brother was a king among kings. Nobody could ever take his place."

I stopped moving and turned to him. "That shouldn't stop you from stepping up."

He shook his head. "No. I mean, yes. I do want to be king. And yes, I want your backing. But that ain't the only reason I'm here."

The men on the council wouldn't consider the women's opinions. If Robert was there to ask for my support, it was out of respect to his brother. I knew the thought of me ruling the kingdom hadn't dared enter his mind.

"You going to make a good king, Robert. Not that it matter, but I believe in you. I know William would be proud of you."

"Thank you, Luella."

"So what's the other reason you here?"

He scratched his head. "I just wanted to come by and tell you that you been a fine queen. If they make me king, you don't got to move out this palace. I'll stay where I'm at."

"Nonsense. The king belongs in the palace. Any wife will expect it."

"Wife?"

"Don't you plan to marry soon?"

"Well, I ain't exactly attached to nobody at the moment."

"That'll change. Now get on over to that clearing and make your case to them men about who our next king ought to be."

I turned to pour him a cup of water from the pitcher on the table, but then I heard the feet of the chair scrape on the floor and suddenly he was gone.

THIRTEEN

I couldn't help myself. Neither could Jola. We hid in the trees,
just out of the men's line of sight. After they'd settled all the
other business, they turned to the matter of leadership. The
sounds of the children shouting reached the clearing. Between
them and the rustling of leaves, it was hard to hear.

"To King William," said Hal. I knew all the men on the council
and not just by their voices. William had not kept council delib-
erations from me, freely sharing what men said during the meetings, asking my opinion when he was conflicted. I knew what each
man valued, what things was important to them.

Though the king and queen enjoyed the trappings of royalty,
the kingdom was set up so that the council made decisions as a
group. The king led the meetings, but he made no decisions on his
own. We didn't set a number for the council. It was our most
trusted group—a small number could read, others was known for
the high worth of their labor, while others had survived horrors

that commanded our respect. Now that William was gone, the council numbered eight.

"Brothers, I think it ain't no surprise to you that I'm here asking to be your king. Course we didn't plan for this day. My brother, William, is a good man. He helped us build this place from nothing. He led us here."

"You heard from him?"

I strained to listen, wondering if there was more news Robert hadn't shared with me.

"Just that his eyes ain't come back. He still at the rooming house and the other men seeing to him, making sure he eat. He ain't in the best of spirits, but that's to be expected."

There was some chatter, and I could hear that the news was disturbing to them. Maybe they had been expecting his return, just like I had.

Robert continued, his voice rising above the others. "When we talk about Africa, we ain't talking about one thing. We talking about all the things our people used to know over there. We talking about different tongues and ways. But one thing we always knew was that we lived a life in that other land across the ocean before we was brought here in the dark of ships and worked to death. So we made something here on this mountain, something to remind us of who we used to be before they tried to kill us."

Jola poked me, her eyes wide in surprise. Robert was talking in a way neither of us had ever heard. Holding court even. His voice didn't carry the deep tones of his brother's, but he was loud and clear above the wind. And from the silence surrounding him, I could tell the men was listening.

"We got to finish what my brother started. We got to keep on keeping on, away from the Klan and the U.S. government and all the lies they tell us. We got to be free!"

A single shout rose up from the men, and although I couldn't see their faces and didn't linger long enough to hear them take an actual vote, I knew Robert would be our next king.

WHEN THE WOMEN traveled together, nobody bothered us. Most everybody knew us as the kingdom women on account of how we wore them shawls. When we got to town, one of us would go in the store and purchase what was needed. Afterward, we'd push the cart carrying our things back up the hill.

On one of our shopping days, when one of the women complained of her knee hurting, we began discussing various remedies among ourselves.

Wrap it in leaves.

Go to the creek. The water will loosen you right up.

A compress will do wonders.

I got some roots I can put on it. Dried 'em out and brung 'em with me up the mountain.

"You all just stay put," I said to the women. "I'll go inside and ask what they got for it. We go up and down that hill so much, I'm not surprised about that knee."

Mr. Frank didn't like me browsing about the store. He preferred that I come to him at the counter and tell him what I needed. Then he would pick out the items for me. He was happy to do business with the kingdom, he always said. Besides, the Widow vouched for us.

"Good day, Mr. Frank."

"Well, hello, Luella. What brings you in here today?"

"Just two bags of grain."

"Sure thing. That's all?"

I pointed at the cabinet of medicines. "I was hoping to get something to rub on a knee."

"You cut yourself?"

"No, just a knee feeling bad is all."

"You're going to have to wait for the apothecarist to come around. We're all out of everything. He come once a month or so."

"The what?"

"Apothecarist. That's the man that bring the medicine and such."

"Hmm," I said. I still hadn't caught the word, but I figured he meant something like the white folks' root worker. "Okay, I'll just take that grain. And you got any cloth today?"

"I sure do. Some fine cotton muslin right here." He unfolded a dull piece of fabric. I thought of the colors we could dye it.

"I'll give you a good price for it, too," he said.

I reached out to touch it, but he pulled it just out of my reach.

"I'll take it," I said.

He wrote up a ticket and brought the grain outside to load in our cart. I passed the fabric to one of the women.

As we walked through the town, I was thinking of the remedies the women had suggested. These women had brought all that knowledge up here with them. Why couldn't we put together something for a knee?

We made our way back up the hill, and as the women chatted, I remained quiet, thinking. Maybe we could make a liniment. All kinds of plants and roots grew on the mountain. Surely we could work something up just from God's earth.

I mentioned my liniment idea to the women, and they said they could do it. We didn't have no root workers in the kingdom yet, but that didn't mean we couldn't see about the sick. One woman had made tinctures back at the home place. Most of us knew how to ferment one thing or another.

"Selling mean it's got to be better than other liniments," said Rachel. "And people got to want to buy it from us."

"Maybe the Widow Davis could offer it to guests at the inn," suggested Jola.

I smiled at my friend. She always stood behind my ideas, ready to help. We'd already had our first frost and would have to wait until spring, when the plants offered up their treasures. Plenty of time.

I couldn't wait to tell Robert. I was still getting to know him, still figuring out differences between him and his brother, but one thing I knew for sure was that Robert was an easy man. Add to it, this was a better idea than soap and it sure wasn't hooch.

Later that evening, while he was eating his dinner on the steps outside the cabin that he shared with three other men, I approached and laid my idea out to him. "The women want to make a liniment. Sell it to the travelers that come up the turnpike. And in town. And maybe at the inn."

"The Widow's son running the inn now. He ain't like his mama." He looked up at me from the step, as if surprised that I'd suddenly appeared during mealtime and thrust this idea on him.

He was right. I'd been around the son just twice, but I'd seen how he fancied himself smarter than he was. "What about travelers on the turnpike. Like at that watering hole where they stop to let the horses drink. We could set up there. And we could push a cart through town and sell right off the cart. Maybe even stop at folks' houses."

He didn't say nothing, and I could see him turning it over.

"If we grow a reputation for the good stuff, there could be a nice penny to be made," I added.

"Everybody do got pains, especially the railroad workers."

"All we got to get is some jars. Mr. Frank at the store could get us some. He always give me a fair price."

"The men too busy to help. Can the women handle all this without us? Selling it, too?"

"Have you seen how much work these women do? They canned so much fruit this winter it almost filled the storehouse."

"And the money go to the treasury?"

I nodded. "Course. Ain't we part of this settlement same as y'all?"

"Y'all need a house to work. We can build you one."

"You will?"

"And a schoolhouse, too."

I watched him carefully as he ate his food. "You know I asked William about a schoolhouse, don't you."

He was silent for so long, I thought I'd guessed wrong. I wondered if he knew how William was with me, the way he spat words sometimes.

Then I heard Robert say without looking up at me, "I love my brother, Luella. But I ain't him. I hope you know that by now."

I didn't say nothing in return.

ROBERT WAITED FOR the next meeting of the council to propose the idea to the men about the liniment. He made the case that there was enough women now to set aside their duties. A regular trio of women cooked. Two women was learning the little ones. Two more worked in the inn, and three sewed and mended. This new group, he told them, would work on creating the best liniment the Carolinas had ever seen.

I didn't hear him say none of this, but he told me later in detail, sharing the few objections that arose. If the women mixed up the liniment, would they sell it, too? Who else was selling it down in the town, and would they be upset? But he said there wasn't no protests, just men thinking out loud. Then they moved on to what the kingdom could do with the money. Like add another room to some houses and buy tools for work. With the growing community, we needed more seed to feed the people.

In the end, the money decided it. We needed more of it, plain and simple.

Once Robert gave me the word, I handpicked the women who would help me. Jola. Eliza. Rachel. The first thing we needed was to buy the alcohol, then figure out a mixture. The liniment would contain alcohol mixed with an herb. The cook from Widow Davis's inn had told me about a plant that grew on the mountain. She called it *seng*. She said it was the thing that would set our liniment apart. We all knew we needed to make ours better than the others.

"Some liniments warm and some cool," Rachel said to us. "What y'all got in mind?"

"Back home, we used comfrey," said Jola.

"I don't trust this *seng* business," piped up Eliza. I'd chosen her because once we made these decisions, she would outwork all of us put together. I sometimes wondered when Eliza slept.

She continued. "Maybe we give them what they used to 'stead of trying to change things."

"I agree with Eliza," said Rachel. "I say we make what everybody used to, but we sell it cheap."

"Cheap," I repeated. I wanted to lead, but William had taught me that in order to lead, I had to listen first. "Hmm, okay. Let's try it with comfrey and see if it sell. If it don't, we talk again."

Our first decision was what would we name it. We knew we would need to give it a label so when folks asked for it by name, they knew where to find it. It didn't take much deliberation. We would call it Happy Land Liniment.

Now all we had to do was wait until spring.

WE DECIDED TO work at Eliza's until the men could finish our house. Unlike some of the families, Eliza and Hal lived in one of the old cabins with only one room for their living. Even though Hal sat on the council, they had no children and preferred one room because it was easier to warm. We uncovered the windows to help with the sting of the alcohol scent and lined up the jars. One of us poured the alcohol while another scooped herbs into the jar. Once the jars was almost full, the third woman capped and shook. The mixtures would have to sit for weeks before they was ready. After the mixture settled, we would strain out the herbs, leaving the liquid behind.

After Hal left each day, three of us arrived at the house to set up for work.

"It's been months. Your husband ain't coming back?" Rachel asked me directly. Even Jola, my friend since we was babies, didn't push me too hard on William's absence. I knew my confidences was safe with Jola. If she did share secrets, I trusted she would shape them with love and not cause trouble. But this was Eliza's house, and I had to mark my words.

"I don't think so," I said.

"They say he blind. That true?" Rachel pressed.

"That's what they say."

"Leave her alone," said Jola. "You don't see nobody asking you about that old man you sneaking around with."

"What old man?'

"Both of y'all hush," Eliza said.

I passed Rachel three more empty jars and she lined them up on the table. I picked up the jug of alcohol and began to pour.

"I ain't asking nothing that everybody else ain't wondering," Rachel said. Even though she was still young, she'd lost four children and then her husband to fever, and though she was still young enough to bear more, she refused to start another family. If there was one thing I had learned during slavery, it was that hope was a fragile thing.

"I will say," Eliza began carefully, "everybody still consider you queen."

I looked at her. "But I'm not."

"The kingdomfolk say different. You still living in the palace."

"Until Robert take a wife."

"The day I take another husband will be the day that man take a wife," Rachel snapped. "Which means to say never."

"Luella." Eliza's voice was serious, and I was listening. "I believe the women want to talk to you."

"What you mean?"

"I mean they got concerns, and they believe you the one to listen."

I tried to think of how I might listen to them. One by one?

That would take a while. Call a meeting? I'd never done that before. Would they even come? And what would I say? William would not have approved of me convening the women. He would've said they needed to go to the council. The community only worked if we stayed as one.

But Eliza was not known for wasting words. If she was advising me to meet with them, the rumblings was real.

Jola continued to work. "Let's put rosemary in these."

"Alright, I'll talk to them." I made a decision. It wasn't no need to consult Robert. I would gather the women that evening. "Put out the word for the women to meet me at the creek just before sunset, before the dinner hour."

"That soon?" Jola stopped what she was doing when I said that.

"Yes. And can you gather up some wildflowers? I want to give the women gifts."

Jola nodded. "Will y'all be fine here without me? I better start getting the word out."

I had no idea what I would say to the women once we was all together, but I could feel my blood coursing. Just the prospect of gathering the women together had done something to me.

FOURTEEN

J ola put the word out and they came. And though I didn't
count, I could see with my eyes that nearly all the women
showed up. Some carried babies tied across their backs. A few
wore pants—for there was women among us who worked alongside the men. The cooks still wore their aprons tied across their
fronts. It was just before the evening meal, and we had interrupted
their preparations. Still, they came.

The women encircled me, and I froze up, not knowing exactly
what to say. I'd called the meeting impulsively, risked the council's
ire when they found out. Jola had tied bunches of the flowers into
bundles. She'd worked with the quickness of youth and was now
walking around, passing them out. It had taken her nearly an hour,
but as I watched the women put the flowers to their noses, I knew
it had been worth it.

Pleased by their gifts, the women turned their attention to
me, curiosity as to why I'd called the meeting burning on their
faces. So I inhaled and tried to quiet my nerves by saying, "Ladies."

The word was a powerful one for us. Ladyhood had been a term reserved for white women. So when I said it, they heard it. It was hard not to examine every word in these days of freedom. We'd always known the power of language, in some ways more powerful than the whip, but it was during freedom that we took back our words, starting with what we called ourselves.

"I brought you here today to talk to you about the changes you been seeing in the kingdom. As y'all know, my husband, William, was hurt down at the mines."

I didn't use a fancy voice. They wouldn't appreciate me putting on airs. But I sure wished I could talk like the Montgomery brothers. Now, them men could say some words!

"William ain't coming back, and now Robert our king. I don't come to you out of no disrespect for neither one of them."

The women began to murmur, but I kept talking. "But I hear tell that y'all still think I'm queen. Thank you for that honor, undeserving as I am."

My humility was genuine; if it wasn't, the women would sense it. They listened calmly, waiting to hear what else I might say.

"Now, I know what y'all thinking. William ain't dead, and I ain't no widow. But he might as well be. I know it's a few of y'all that had a man leave you during slavery. Ain't nothing worse. It's like they dead, ain't it."

They was quiet. I'd touched on a pain few wanted to speak of.

"What I really want y'all to know is this. I didn't ask to be queen. I just wanted to come here and build a new life, same as you. But God had a path for me, and I followed that path. I'm still the same Luella, a girl come up from South Carolina, a girl whose mama died bringing me into this world, a girl who had to find my own way."

I paused, trying to figure out how to end my little speech.

"King Robert a good king for us. And if there is something y'all want me to take him, I'm happy to do it. Just holler."

I had never gone to them like that. We was a community, and the men on the council acted in the interest of all of us. No one had ever gone to the women and asked what we wanted. We'd always believed the needs of the kingdom was same as everybody's needs.

But what did us women desire in freedom times? Ain't nobody had ever thought to ask us. The things we been through and seen was different than it was for the men. And even in the times that it was the same, we didn't have a say in how we could fix it. And that didn't make no kind of sense.

They said nothing at first. Just looked at me like I had grown a second nose. Finally, one of the women spoke. Margaret was the wife of Reverend Couch, who had brought us many of our new kingdom residents.

"We need a place to work. A cabin for the women to sew together and make this new liniment I been hearing about. The cookhouse too busy. And most of us doing all this work outside when the weather permit or dirtying up our own cabins. In winter it ain't easy. Everybody ain't got a big house like you."

Jola and I exchanged looks. Margaret was right, but she didn't know the work house was coming. Robert and the council had decided on it. Before I could answer, another voice rang out.

"I want a pretty dress. You call us ladies, but I don't feel like none. We work all week but it be nice to have a Sunday dress. The liniment is going to sell and we all know it. Can't we get some nice cloth with the money from the treasury?"

I heard some affirmations from the group. Everybody was nodding in agreement.

"Alright, alright—" I began.

"We do the cooking so we ought to have a say in the seed for crops. Why only the men go to market for seed? Every year it's the same . . ."

"I hear you. We can talk about all this. Let me talk to the king."

"The king! We need a seat on the council, Miss Luella." It was Margaret again. "You ain't even invited to them meetings and you the queen!"

With that, the meeting erupted and I couldn't get their attention. The women began to walk away, their disgruntled voices casting aside all order. We'd run out of time. The men would be back soon, and it would be time to hit the mealtime drum. I moved among them, touching arms, addressing the ladies by name.

I would have to tell Robert about this gathering soon as he finished work for the day, about the women's demands, before word reached him through somebody else.

I DIDN'T HAVE much time. All across the settlement women carried dinner back to their cabins from the cookhouse. Others delivered plates to the cabins housing the elderly or uncoupled. After the meal, the children picked up the serving bowls from front porches and ran them down to the creek to be washed before returning them to the cookhouse.

To my surprise, before I could find him, Robert showed up at the palace with a gift meant to surprise me. I hadn't known he had been down the turnpike that day. Robert recounted how he had managed a trade with a man. Well-sharpened tools in exchange for this mule who was looking at me out of doleful eyes.

"You can ride her if you want," he was saying excitedly. "The man say she won't even buck. You want to name her?"

I looked at Robert skeptically. "A name?" I'd never had a mule of my own before, and I'd sure never named an animal. I knew mules couldn't have babies, and I wondered if she carried the same sadness I did.

"You could call her Legs 'cause she got some long legs. I ain't seen legs this long on a mule never."

I reached out to the animal and placed a hand on her muzzle. She leaned into me as if for a scratch. No, she wasn't sad. Somebody had loved on this animal, and now she was looking at me to do the same.

"Delight."

"What's that?"

"I think I'll call her Delight," I said.

He clapped his hands loudly. "Now, that's a name! See, I knew you'd like her. Dee-light!"

He was still chuckling to himself, pleased with his own generosity.

Wish me luck, Delight. Us women going need it.

"Do you want to come inside? I can call for one of the women to send your dinner here," I told him as he tied the mule to the post.

I called out to one of the children running past and asked him to bring the king's dinner to the palace. Once we was inside, I motioned to the chair where William used to sit and picked up the water pitcher. "Food ought to be here in a minute. You want some water?"

"Do you like the mule? Or you just pretending?" He splashed his hands in the bowl and wiped them on a rag.

121

"It seem nice," I said truthfully. "But I don't know why you traded your tools. Far as I can tell, this animal don't seem like much of a worker."

"Because I wanted to see you happy again." He set his eyes on me seriously, and when I tried to smile, he didn't return the mirth. I was so glad when the young boy knocked on the door with his plate. I set it on the table beside his cup of water.

Unlike William, Robert ate quickly and without speaking much. On his plate, I placed extra peppers from the patch I kept beside the palace. I had already observed that Robert liked his food spicy, while William had a hankering for salt. I knew I needed to stop comparing Robert to his brother, but I couldn't help myself.

"I spoke with the women today."

He barely looked up. "Which women?"

"All of them."

He glanced up at me, and when he saw my expression, he put down his fork. "You got something to tell me."

"I got something to ask."

"Go right ahead."

"They was asking for a meeting. Hal Whitmire's wife, Eliza, told me so."

He nodded once.

"I didn't think it would be much of nothing, but they had some things to say."

"What things?"

I decided to start with the biggest request. I understood a little about Robert, and one thing I knew was he didn't like to tarry.

"They want a seat on the council."

He wiped his mouth with his sleeve. Then he took a sip of his water. I could tell he was thinking.

"They want a say in the seeds we buy for crops. They say it's the same every year. And they want fabric for dresses." I spoke fast, then exhaled once I'd uttered the last.

"And they think they need a seat on the council in order to make these things happen?"

I nodded.

"But why not just ask you? You could always ask me and I could take it to the men. Ain't that easier? Everybody think you still queen, anyhow."

So he knew this, too. How had I not known that they thought of me this way? "Funny you say that. The women also think it's a shame I don't have a seat on the council and I'm the queen."

"Luella, what's this all about? Are you stirring up trouble?"

"Why you think this is trouble?"

"I'm just trying to figure out where you coming from."

"I ain't got nothing to hide. If I wanted a seat on the council, I would've asked for it long ago." That wasn't entirely true. William hadn't been the kind of man I would have dared say such a thing to. I wasn't even sure I would have brought any of the women's demands to him.

Robert settled back in his chair. "I'll have to take it to the men. This won't be my decision to make and you know it."

"Mind if I say one more thing?"

"Ain't no choice in the matter, is it."

"Ask for two seats."

"Now, that is you, ain't it."

I nodded. "I don't want to be the only woman on that council if it comes to it. Ain't no honor in that."

He picked his fork back up. His face was soft, and I knew he would do his best.

"Hey. You think I could try riding Delight after dinner?" I asked.

He looked up at me and smiled. "Wouldn't nothing make me happier, Queen Lu."

And the way he looked at me, I knew, sure as there was a God, that he was a different man than William, despite their common blood.

FIFTEEN

Nikki

Mother Rita promised Maddie Mae would help me get ready for flower market, but she never gave me the neighbor's phone number. I would just have to stop by Maddie Mae's house unannounced. It seems rude, but maybe that's just how they do it here. Miss Maddie Mae. I don't even know what to respectfully call her. I try to wrap my head around Southern courtesies.

She lives just half a mile down the road from Mother Rita, but it's not walkable because there are no sidewalks. Her house is neat and tidy, the front drive covered in small pebbles that crunch under the tires of my rental Honda. Out front her flower beds are enclosed by miniature fences. Mother Rita mentioned deer. I wonder how Maddie Mae keeps them out.

Before I get out of the car, she appears on the porch, as if she has been expecting me.

"Hello there, young lady!" she calls out.

"Sorry to drop by," I say as I get out of the car. "I didn't have your phone number."

"Oh, you don't need to call. As long as my car in the driveway, you can stop by anytime. If I don't answer the door, I'm in the bath. Just wait out here on the porch until I can get to you."

Inside, her house is cluttered, a lifetime of bric-a-brac lining every surface. She collects Black dolls, some of them in fine dresses with carefully curled hair, others historical representations of Black women wearing head rags and aprons. A glass-enclosed credenza is crammed with dolls of every size. One shelf is devoted to couples, men and women decked out in similar finery. I peer through the glass.

"How long have you been collecting?"

"I started as a child, but it was hard to find nice Black dolls back then. So every time I find one I like, I buy it. Some of these dolls you'll never find again. My daddy used to bring them back from his travels."

"Your daddy traveled?"

"Oh, yes. Daddy was in the navy. He served his country in two wars, yes sir, he did. He and my mama grew up together right here in Hendersonville, but Daddy was always a born traveler. He wasn't happy unless he was stepping foot on a ship or train. So after his service, he became a cook for a businessman from Asheville who traveled all the time. Mama was happy right here. She kept the house for us three kids so when Daddy came home everything was in good order. Kids clean and presentable. Hot meals. Clothes pressed. Mama kept a strict house, yes sir, she did."

There isn't a speck of dust on any of the dolls. Maddie Mae's house might be cluttered, but she takes care with it.

"You want something to drink? You ate today?"

"I ate already, but—"

"How about some shortbread and iced tea? My grandson, Stephen, got a sweet tooth, so I bake up something once a week. You like shortbread cookies? I mean, don't everybody?"

"Yes, ma'am."

"You gluten free?"

"No, ma'am." I can't hide my surprise.

"What y'all think up in D.C., that we're a bunch of hillbillies? We know all about allergies and food intolerance. We got a nice Ingles supermarket that's got everything in it you could imagine. You been there yet? Rita been a vegetarian for years and she can even cook vegan if she want to." She disappears into the kitchen.

"No, ma'am, course I don't think y'all hillbillies," I call from the living room.

"You stick around for a while and you'll get to know us. You've stayed away too long as it is. Time to get to know your people. Come on back in the kitchen!"

Her forthrightness reminds me of Mother Rita. No wonder they're such good friends. The kitchen is airy, but just as cluttered as the living room. The counter space is covered with various appliances—a stand mixer, toaster, slow cooker, bread machine. In the middle of the kitchen, eight chairs surround a long wooden table. On the table sits a ceramic African American lady with her arms wrapped around a basket that holds a pile of real mandarins.

"Sit down, sit down."

I sit and glance out the back window into a brightly lit backyard. I have been feeling overwhelmed today, still processing the news of Mother Rita's illness, but Maddie Mae's kitchen soothes me.

"How's Rita doing?" she asks. "Bryan texted me this morning."

"She's doing better. Just dehydrated. They're getting some

fluids in her. She ought to be able to come home in the next day or so. I took her some soup and corn bread." I try to sound cheery, but Mother Rita looked thin and tired when I visited.

"You look just like your mama, you know."

I catch her staring at me. A kettle sits over a fire on the stove, and the heat is beginning to warm the kitchen. My nose is moist with sweat and I wipe it.

"You knew my mama?"

"Oh, yes. I've known your family since I was a little girl. Rita and I grew up together."

"Miss Maddie Mae," I begin.

"No need for the *Miss*. Just call me Maddie."

"Yes, ma'am." I tack on the *ma'am*. "Maddie, can I ask you a question?"

"Course you can."

"What happened between my mama and grandmama? I don't really understand why they stopped speaking."

Maddie Mae pauses before responding. "What did they tell you?"

"Nothing. It was like a door slammed shut."

"You know, your mama was never built for this town. I think she felt suffocated by it. She was out of here on the first thing smoking. I think that hurt Rita worse than anything. So when they actually did have a big kerfuffle, years later, all it took were a few words."

The kettle starts to whistle, and she shuts off the heat.

"But what was the kerfuffle all about?" I ask, borrowing her old-fashioned word.

"Child, don't start me lying. I don't know the whole story."

I sit quietly, hoping she'll say more if I don't respond. I guess correctly.

"All I know is that it had something to do with the land. They had a big argument about it."

Something to do with the land. Mother Rita had said it all started with Luella. The kingdom is the preamble to her revealing what she promised—why she and Mama don't speak. She thinks I need to know about Luella first. I just don't understand what all this has to do with Mama. She hasn't lived in Hendersonville in over forty years.

Maddie Mae pauses. "Rita is my best friend, but she was always tight-lipped when it came to her family. I don't think in all the years I knew her and Herbert she ever said one unkind word about him. And don't you think every couple have an argument or two over sixty years of marriage?"

"I don't remember Granddaddy Herbert. Besides, I always imagined couples like them didn't argue much. Not like me and my ex."

Maddie Mae takes my hands in hers. "You know what my mama told me once? The only difference between a married couple and a divorced couple is that one of them decided to stay."

I smile a little. Maddie Mae is a gentle soul. I wonder if she is like me, one of the ones who decided *not* to stay. I see no evidence of a husband in the house, and though she has a grandson, it doesn't mean she ever married.

She places a plate of cookies on the table, peeling back the plastic wrap as she speaks. "You stick around a while, maybe you can get it all out of her. I've probably already spoken more than I should."

My lip quivers. "I leave Sunday."

She pauses to stare at me. "Why the rush? This is your first visit here, and now you want to rush off."

"My daughter is staying alone without me. And I have a listing I need to sell. I'm a real estate agent."

"I thought your daughter had graduated high school already. And don't y'all sell houses online these days?"

"That's true. My ex-husband is helping out with the property. He works in my office."

"Well, look at God." She smiles. "Here. Take a cookie. The tea will be ready in a minute, and we got to talk about these flowers."

"Yes, ma'am," I say, though the flowers are the furthest thing from my mind.

MADDIE MAE MEETS me at sunrise the next day. We'll do all the cutting ourselves. I wear Mother Rita's clean apron over my T-shirt and jeans and lace up my new boots so my shoestrings won't flop. It's a crisp July morning, the sky foggy, though I know it'll burn off by afternoon. The forecast is sunny with a chance of more sun.

"Don't look so nervous," Maddie Mae says, setting her coffee mug down on Mother Rita's kitchen counter.

"I just don't want to mess this up."

"You cleaned the buckets last night and wiped down the clippers like I told you?"

"Yes, ma'am," I say. "I used the detergent and a little bleach in the water."

"Since it's your first time, we'll keep it simple."

"We've got to cut and make arrangements, right?"

"Yes, I'll get you started cutting, and once we fill a few buckets, I'll go to the shed and start arranging."

"Do customers ever ask you to make an arrangement on-site?" I don't know the first thing about how to fill out a bouquet.

"Sometimes. You'll get the hang of it in no time."

"You make it sound so easy. I still can't believe you and Mother Rita do all this by yourselves."

She takes a sip of her coffee. "Why? Because we're senior citizens? We been working our whole lives. Unless this old hip gives out, I reckon I could still climb this mountain if I had to."

"I'd rather climb the mountain than sell these flowers," I say.

A young man carries a folding table into the kitchen. "I brought this extra table because the leg was broken on the other one."

"This is my grandson, Stephen. He's seventeen."

Facial hair spreads across his chin in patches. "Morning," he greets us quietly.

I follow the two of them outside, tapping Mother Rita's stick loudly on the ground.

"Child, what are you doing?" Maddie Mae asks.

"I'm scared of snakes," I say, hoping to gain some sympathy.

She laughs. "Girl, ain't no snakes!"

"Just watch your step," Stephen warns.

"What do I do if I see one?"

"Run!" Maddie Mae is still laughing at me.

"Oh, I'm going to do more than run," I say. "They're going to hear me hollering all the way in South Carolina."

"I'll kill it if you see one." Stephen puffs up his chest. "Last summer, I—"

"You hush up." Maddie Mae shoots him a look. "Ain't no snakes."

The breeze sweeps over me. There's a lean, hungry look to the sky, as if it still needs to fill itself with the day. I place the shears in the pocket of my apron and push the cart behind Maddie Mae. She opens the gate and moves swiftly down the line, looking through the flowers. I'm not sure what she's looking for, so I follow.

"Just trying to decide what's ready," she says. "Rita did a real good job cleaning everything up."

Stephen enters the shed, and I hear him turning on the air-conditioning units.

"Let me cut a few for you to get you started. Look-a-here." She takes a flower in her left hand and snips it with her right. "I'm guessing you've cut a flower before and know to cut the stem on an angle like so."

"Yes, ma'am." Mama taught me that. She doesn't have a garden, but she does keep a vase of fresh flowers on her kitchen table. I remember how she takes her time in the supermarket floral department, picking the freshest blossoms. The more I think about it, the more I realize my mama does have a practiced hand with arranging flowers. Had all the signs of my family story been right in front of me all along and I just hadn't known?

"Some flowers you cut while they're still buds. Others you have to wait until they open. If you cut some of them while they're still budding, they won't open," Maddie Mae is saying.

"How do you know which is which?"

"You learn. Come on."

We walk down the row, and she explains everything to me.

"Once we get to market, how do we price everything?" I ask.

She shakes her shoulders impatiently. I wish Shawnie were here with me. She loves chatting with strangers and would enjoy this whole flower market experience. I try to remember the last time she and I did something like this together, just the two of us.

Stephen emerges from the shed, carrying poles for the tent.

Maddie Mae's voice rings out evenly across the rows. "Flowers can be grown from bulbs or tubers or stems or seeds. Usually the bulbs bloom earliest."

"Like tulips?"

"That's right. Now, when you sell at market, you have to think about what looks good in a bouquet. Rita grows these snapdragons to give a little drama. The amaranth give a unique look. Look over there. The black-eyed Susans are nice."

"That's a lot to think about." I need more coffee.

"You get used to it. Now, to get the nicest flowers on the day you harvest, there's a lot of preparation involved. When you come out here in the morning, the last thing you want to do is have to pick through a bunch of dead blossoms. So Rita and I do a lot of deadheading, grooming, staking, and cleaning up beforehand. But we enjoy it. Keep you young."

"How often do you turn on the sprinklers?" I look for sprinkler heads in the ground.

"Sprinklers? Girl, we ain't that fancy. Besides, it rains enough here. We might water every once in a while during a dry spell. Then we just pull that hose out over yonder. Don't need no sprinklers."

As she cuts, she carefully places the flowers in the bucket. "You hold the flower with one hand and cut with the other. Now, after you cut, you want to strip off the leaves from the bottom of the stem, like this. That makes the arrangement pretty and keeps the leaves from sullying the water."

She cuts several flowers and strips them before placing them in the bucket.

"Go ahead and try it."

I cut a flower, but when I strip the foliage from the base, I pull too close and scrape my fingers.

"Where are your gloves? Stephen, bring Nikki some gloves! Now, once we fill this first set of buckets, my grandson will take them in the shed so they can stay cool while we finish the rest."

"How many buckets we plan to fill?"

"Not that many. Like I say, we'll keep it simple today. We just don't want to miss the market, because Rita got regulars. They get their flowers from her every single week."

While I wait for the gloves, I take a peek at my phone out of habit, though it's too early for messages. I am missing my mama so much right now. I'd give anything to have her and Shawnie out here in this garden with me, basking in Maddie Mae's attention just as I am. I put my phone in my pocket and try to focus. All is quiet, as if nature is holding its breath to see what damage I cause to this pristine garden. The short chirps of a warbler erupt from a nearby tree, breaking the quiet. I startle but manage to catch its flutter as it takes flight.

I imagine Luella walking these hills, planning what she might grow each season and how much. Whether Mother Rita's story about a royal queen and king is true or not, I know Luella made a home on this mountain along with other freedpeople. I wonder what life was like for them, how difficult it must have been to make a life in those days. According to the Bobo record, Luella would have been born around 1850 and spent fifteen years enslaved. After all she'd been through, it must have been quite a leap of imagination to call herself a queen.

Mother Rita got her love of flowers from her mother, who must have gotten it from her mother and grandmother. Yet another locked door of secrets. Answers to questions I hadn't even realized I had. In the last row, Mother Rita has planted tall stalks of pale blue blossoms that make me think *glamour*. The show-offs of the garden. Y'all think you cute, don't you? I laugh and catch myself. I cannot talk to these flowers like Mother Rita does.

I read the signs staked in the garden, identifying the flowers.

How frustrating to be out here and not know the names of things. It strikes me that the naming of God's creations is important work, just like the naming of human beings. I think again of the nameless rocks in my family cemetery up the hill.

"Miss Maddie, my grandmother says our family lost this land and doesn't own it anymore. Do you know anything about that?"

Maddie bends over to pick up the gloves, as if I haven't just asked her a question. But I know she heard me. "Here, put those gloves on. We got work to do," she says.

SIXTEEN

Luella

We had two seats on the council, and now the women treated me different, waving at me as I walked by, leaving gifts on my porch. Every now and then, a woman would appear at my door with a request. *Queen Luella*, they'd begin, *I got something to ask of you. My boy ain't feeling too good and don't seem to be getting better. You reckon there's money for a proper doctor?* Every meeting, I made a new request, and I wasn't shy about it. Women wanted an accounting of the treasury. They wanted to sit down for a while after birthing. They wanted spices for cooking, paid "information wanted" notices in the papers to find missing family. The women had turned a corner, and we wasn't going back. Things had changed, and everybody could feel it.

Soon after we got our seats on the council, the men finished building our house. We finally had a roof over our heads for making the liniment and sewing and weaving and so forth. Jola, Rachel, Eliza, and I chose a day when we could place our bottles on the shelves. I met the women there, carrying a bag full of bottles that clinked as I walked.

"We need to send the children out to pick us some more herbs. I think we running low."

"Luella, what was your idea on what to mix in the liniment?" asked Eliza.

We had been using comfrey. But ginseng grew all over the mountain, and I knew some of its properties—it helped with swelling and could pull the fever out. It was springtime, and the herb was flourishing on the mountain. The deer loved to eat the seeds, and they would drop them all through the woods, causing fresh seng to spring up in new places each year. Our supply was nearly endless.

"Ginseng," I said.

"Rattlesnakes hide in them patches," grumbled Rachel.

"Be quiet," Eliza snapped. "We could try it. What else, Luella?"

A lot of folks thought a liniment was supposed to stink, trading in a belief that the worse it smelled, the better it worked. But I thought we might choose different. When they rubbed our liniment into their shoulders, feet, arms, legs, back, not only would it make them feel better but a good scent would lift their spirits.

"I say we add some sassafras, too."

"What for?" Jola asked.

"To make it smell nice? Queen Luella, you onto something!" Eliza exclaimed.

"I suppose that is a good idea. Ain't nothing worse than going to bed at night stinking to high heaven," Rachel admitted.

I knew why the women was asking my opinion again. I'd helped them get the council seats, and their respect for me had grown. If I could make this liniment a success, that would earn even more of their trust.

We decided to finish up with our old way of making the liniment, using up all the comfrey we'd already picked. And we would begin to harvest the ginseng, with the help of the children.

Things was looking up in the kingdom.

I HAD BEEN inviting Robert to eat with me at the end of the day, as much to keep me company as to talk about the liniment and plans for the kingdom. That evening was no different. We was eating together so much, the children knew to bring his dinner to the palace. "Y'all men done a good job with the new house. It's space enough for six women to work. We just need a couple more chairs and it be just fine."

I picked up his empty plate, chattering on. "Mr. Frank asked for twenty-five jars to keep in the store at all times. He say our liniment selling better than everything else he got. Say his customers can't get enough of it."

Robert didn't say nothing, but I could feel his eyes on my back. He had been quietly watching me all evening, his eyes steady and focused. My body warmed underneath that stare, but I just kept on talking. "You think we ought to make a tincture, too, or just stick to liniment? We got plenty room to make more. Plenty room. What you think?"

Suddenly he was behind me, smelling of grass. Sweet grass. A flush swept from my toes up to the top of my head. "Robert—" I whispered.

"Shhh."

If I could have dropped to the floor I would have. Just the closeness of his body made mine shut down. My eyes watered with the effort it took me to keep my knees from buckling. My head could barely get around the thoughts forming into words— *this ain't just innocent teasing this time, Luella.*

He spoke words into my hair, his voice hoarse and raw. "I know I ain't my brother, and I hope I ain't overstepping."

Everything in my body tightened, as if all of my muscles had contracted at once. The front door was half-open, but I couldn't hear nothing outside of it. Not the wind, not the chatter of children, not the clink of plates and forks. Behind my eyelids, I could see William. The way he spoke to me. The way he walked with his head held high. Had I loved him? Had I confused love for something else? If I was being honest with myself, there had been a reason I hadn't walked down to that mine. I could have gone after him, regardless of his wishes. I could have demanded he come back and be a husband to me. But I hadn't.

Robert kissed the nape of my neck, and I tried not to panic. Something inside me threatened to slip out, feelings unspoken and shameful. "Be my queen, Lu."

I turned around, slipping my body out of his grasp, but he didn't step back. He was so close I was still pressed against him. Finally, I found the strength to speak, but the words that came out was too honest, too truthful. "How can I be your queen when I'm still married to your brother? What will they think?"

"My brother gone. And you know he ain't coming back. Everybody know that marriage over. It's been almost a year. You ain't got no more obligation to him."

I had not believed William was gone forever, but somehow

Robert's words made it true. He had left me behind, and I needed to move on. *But they are brothers.* Again, my words spoke what my heart had not allowed itself to feel. "But you young, Robert."

"So is you."

"I mean, you must want children and I ain't been able." I shook my head, but when he kissed my lips I pulled his face to mine. I wanted him as badly as he wanted me. Maybe I always had.

We stayed like that for a long time. Then finally, we stepped back from each other, breathless.

As he walked out of the house, he stopped and turned around in the doorway. "If you say yes, Luella, and the Lord provide the blessing of a baby for us, we celebrate. But no matter what, I swear before God, I won't ask for more than my portion."

ROBERT WAS GIVING me time to consider his proposal, but I couldn't help wondering what people would think. Tongues would wag, and I'd be powerless to stop them. In our world, leaving a husband was as momentous as taking one. In a world where just the act of claiming couplehood was an act of rebellion, these choices was no less the magnitude of birth and death.

There was also the matter of women desiring Robert, and not because they wanted to be queen. With his long legs and kind face, Robert caught the eye just like his brother had. The lonely women among us had no shame about preening before him. Since we'd arrived, Robert had married himself to the work of building the settlement, looking neither left nor right. And we all understood that. But now he was our ruler, and that added another piece to him.

I was not unlike them women. I had glimpsed something behind Robert's eyes before, especially when he looked at me. But

I'd always suspected it was because he reminded me of his brother, like two sides of the same coin. Now I believed he had purposely showed me them sides of him when no one was looking. In William's eyes, I saw raw ambition, a need for attention and respect, a resentment that white men had not honored his intellect. In Robert, I saw an ambition that was not solely in his head, but also in his heart. Robert wanted prosperity for our community. He wanted peace and freedom from the ills of a diseased nation. If he could've walled in the kingdom and cut us off in them hills from the outside world, he would have. He wanted to work and see the fruits of his labor, and rest come Sunday. It was simple to him.

And now I knew he also wanted to spend time with me. Forever time. The kind of time without worry of an end. He aroused a heat in me that William never had. With William, I'd wanted to talk and hear his mind at work. With Robert, I also delighted in our evening conversations—him sharing the problems of the council and me responding with assurance or doubt. But unlike with his brother, there was times my body wouldn't even let me hear the words coming out of Robert's mouth. I could barely think when he got too close, my body was so pulsed with tension. The man did something to me.

I couldn't collect my thoughts with a clear head so I went to see Papa. I hadn't told nobody about Robert's proposal, not even Jola. And unlike William, Robert hadn't gone to my papa to ask for my hand. It was all secret and a little shameful. But when I told Papa about Robert's proposal, he didn't seem too surprised. He sat on the council, so Papa had been one of the elders to vote Robert as king. He knew the Montgomery brothers as well as anybody.

"You ain't saying much, Papa. What you think?"

"What you think, Lu?"

I was having a hard time saying my feelings out loud, even to myself. "I think William a fine man, and I don't want to disrespect him."

"Yes, he is. And Robert?"

"I think he a fine man, too."

Papa's cabin wasn't close to nobody else's, having been built at a bend in the path that wound through the settlement. We was sitting inside, close to the fire. Nobody could hear us, but we still spoke in a hush. It didn't matter, though. I knew if I took Robert as husband, all of this would be out in the open.

"So what you think?" I asked again.

"You know why I never married again after your mama?"

I shook my head.

"Because I was scared. I didn't want to hurt like that ever again."

I'd grown up in the shadow of Papa's grief, and I'd seen him shed many a tear in the dark of our church back in Cross Anchor. But now he spoke with a dry-eyed finality that was filled with more regret than sadness.

"So you telling me not to be scared, ain't you. Even though I'm still married."

He pulled his blanket up over his lap. "The Bible say if the unbelieving depart, let him depart."

"Papa, I think I love him," I whispered.

Then he said to me what I had always known to be true. "If it don't work, there's always a place for you to lay your head in this house." He smiled tenderly, his smooth face glistening in the light.

I DIDN'T GIVE an answer, but Robert just showed up on my doorstep one evening with a bag, as casually as if he was coming by for another meal. I took the bag from him and put his things away without a word. And he sat down in the chair. Just a quiet assumption of his role as king and my own continued role as queen. He did what I couldn't bring myself to do. Made a decision for both of us.

That night, he waited for me in bed. I felt as nervous as a girl as I blew out the candle. The scent of him filled my nose—that unmistakable grassiness, as if he'd rolled around in it. The surface of my skin prickled, the late autumn chill seeping beneath my gown. I lay down, and he placed an arm around me.

"You want the minister?" he whispered.

I hesitated. "I'm still married. I don't think Reverend Couch will do it. And Papa already gave his blessing."

"You need to ask me something?"

I nestled into the crook of his armpit and asked, "Are you sure?"

He lifted my chin. "Luella Montgomery. I give you what little I got. These hands. This body. This—" He tapped his head. "And this." He tapped his chest. "And these." He tapped both upper arms. "I promise I'm going take care of you till the day I die. I won't leave you never. I belong to you."

He said it because he knew I needed to hear it. I couldn't bear it if he left me like his brother had. I could only survive this if he committed. The words had to have meaning this time because William had stood before my papa and God and promised the same thing.

"Robert Montgomery." He pulled me on top of him. I pushed my hands against his chest to raise my head and look at him. "I give you what little I got." I repeated his words. "I promise to you that I will take care of you till the day I die. I won't leave you never. I belong to you."

He inched a hand up my thigh and pulled my gown up and

over my head. I wore nothing beneath it. He stared at my bare chest and I did not shy. It was as if I had loved him forever, as if the marriage to William was some long-ago life. His hands moved up and down the sides of my body, lightly. A warmth spread between my legs. I could not wait even one more breath.

"Shhh . . ." he whispered, as if I had said more.

"Shhh . . ." he said again, and the sounds in the room magnified as if defying his request, the crackling wood popping and hissing, the wind whistling through the beams, the covers rustling, rubbing against my legs.

"Shhh . . ."

And then all was quiet.

SEVENTEEN

Nikki

At the market, we unload the van and begin to set up our booth. One of the men helps Stephen with the tent and tables. Then Stephen goes over to help him out. The sense of community here is palpable, and as Maddie Mae and I drape the vinyl tablecloths on the table, I feel peaceful. Although I'm still nervous about making the bouquets, I'm enjoying this quiet time as the vendors set up.

A baker sets out breads and pastries in plastic wrap. Two women wrapped in crocheted blankets sit near a tree and give out free yarn. A teenager sells homemade mud pies. A man arranges a selection of vegetables on his table, and I can see that he's popular because of the sheer volume of baskets on his tables. A pair of ceramicists set up plates and coffee mugs streaked with a brilliant shade of teal. It's a small market, but the wares are lovely.

Mother Rita has written the flower prices on small chalkboards. The colorful markers she used were the permanent kind, so the numbers are clear and legible. Before Maddie Mae and I can arrange our tables, we have our first customer—a woman from a booth that sells homemade soaps. Maddie Mae and I wear fanny packs around our waists for the money.

We sit in the chairs Stephen has placed behind the table. It's still early, the weather pleasant. Our booth looks good. Hopefully, we'll have a lot of sales. I take a few pictures with my phone and text them to Shawnie. I wait a few minutes, but she doesn't answer.

"Business will pick up," says Maddie Mae.

I look over at her. The woman's silver hair is perfectly curled at the ears and lines the back of her neck. She's the kind of woman who rolls her hair faithfully every night and never fails to wear a protective satin bonnet. Her skin is smooth and unlined, and she wears a pale pink lipstick and small silver hoops in her ears. Her plumpness rounds out her face, and when she smiles small dimples pinch her cheeks.

"Were you ever married, Miss Maddie?"

"Once. He was a two-timer. I put up with it for years, but after I turned fifty, I didn't have the tolerance for it anymore."

I don't know what to say to that. I can't help but think of Darius. Of all the complaints I could make about him, infidelity isn't one of them.

"They say fifty is a big birthday for women," I reply.

"Every decade for a woman matters. How old are you again?"

"I'm about to turn forty."

She hmphs, as if to say *baby*. I may be young to Maddie Mae, who is probably nearly twice my age, but I can already feel this year is a turning point for me. It has been a long time since I walked through a house and got excited about selling it. I've lost my patience for indecisive clients, and I hate the seven-day workweek. But I don't have any idea what else I could do, so I'm stuck.

My aimlessness is probably reflected in Shawnie. She never talks about the future and seems content with the pocket change she earns at the bakery. On weekends, she and her friends visit thrift stores or sit around in the park listening to music. Both of us are just sleepwalking through our days, and I can't help but feel that the reason she can't get it together is because I can't either.

I marvel at these women's ability to create their own version of family. Since the divorce, it has just been me and Shawnie in our two-bedroom apartment, with Mama occasionally sweeping through to keep us organized. I have a few girlfriends, but nobody close. Not like these two senior women in the hills of North Carolina, living in this remote area and not lonely in the least. Even in a major city, I still feel utterly alone.

"I meant what I said earlier. You ought to stay a little while longer, Nikki."

"Well, of course I'll see Mother Rita through this illness. I won't abandon her." The word *abandon* scrapes grit across my tongue. Had my mother abandoned her? I don't think so. She'd done what every young person ought to do—charted her own path. I wonder if Southern mothers feel a particular betrayal when their children go north. I choose my words carefully, not wanting to offend Maddie Mae. "When she comes home from the hospital, I do have to go back to D.C. But I'll come back soon as I sell this house. You never did answer my question about the land. Do you know anything about that?"

"So you're going to leave just like that, huh? Like your grandmother is a tourist stop."

"I said I was coming back." I'm painfully aware her words are meant to cut.

"Sure you are."

"None of y'all will tell me anything!"

We both realize our voices have carried outside the tent and catch ourselves. I look away from her, annoyed that I've momentarily forgotten my manners.

She's right, and I need to just go ahead and admit it. This is like one of those roots trips, where people go back to the home place and try to discover who they are. It isn't like traveling back in time, but it's close as I can get. Now I've learned that my grandmother is sick. I know what it's like to lose somebody, how they disappear from your life forever, the gap left behind. Truth of the matter, I'm scared half to death and I just want to run away.

Maddie Mae is staring at me so hard, I can feel a hole boring into me. I want to wilt under those eyes.

I look around, praying a customer will approach the booth and save me from Maddie Mae's interrogation. But no one comes. It's just me and her, sitting across from each other in a staring contest. I've been around this type of stubbornness my whole life, and if Maddie Mae thought fifty was the age when she couldn't bear her husband anymore, then I have something to say about forty being the age when I can't bear the women in my family anymore.

"When she finds out Mother Rita is dying, it's going to destroy Mama," I whisper.

"Not if you can help it."

I tilt my head in her direction. "Miss Maddie, why should I be the one to sew up this rip?"

I'm tired of everyone playing coy with me. Either Maddie Mae is going to have to give me answers or I'm going to end this conversation right here and now. I stare back at her as hard as I can.

She takes the bait.

"Well, it ain't no business of mine, but I think I'd want to help if my grandmother was being evicted while lying in her sickbed," she says.

My eyes widen. I knew Mother Rita was claiming some kind of rights to the land, but she didn't say anything about an eviction. Now Maddie Mae has said it, and she looks as if she doesn't have a single regret. She has one of those I-said-it-I-meant-it-I'll-always-represent-it looks on her face.

"Now, you march back down that hill this evening and you demand your grandmother give you some answers. And yes, you can tell her I sent you." She folds her arms across her chest.

I am too stunned to speak. My grandmother is being evicted? Is that what Al Thomas had meant by helping her to pack? Does everyone in town know about this eviction?

AS I DRIVE to the hospital, all I can think is: *My grandmother is being evicted from the land where she was born while she is fighting cancer.* Everything is going from bad to worse, and I don't know how to stop the tailspin. I pick up speed in the Honda. I won't allow her to deflect the conversation this time.

When I enter her room, I can tell from the look on her face that Miss Maddie has already warned her that I know. And she's ready to talk.

"Sit," she commands.

Too tired to protest, I sink into the chair beside her bed.

"You ever heard of something called heirs' property?"

"You mean like when heirs make a claim on a title?"

"Something like that. Down here, it's the way a lot of Black folks lose their land. All my life, I've been raised to know what this land meant to my family. The women in my family passed it hand to hand down through the generations. But my mother had an older brother."

"I never knew that."

"Uncle Willie. He had some children, though I never kept in touch with those cousins. They moved away from here long ago."

I consider her phrase *hand to hand*. "Wait, are you about to tell me there was no will?"

"Black folks didn't trust the legal system in those days. Most times, you walked up to a courthouse and you had to pass by a Confederate statue just to enter the front door. It was like they was telling you that you weren't welcome and never would be. It wasn't coincidence that they put those statues in front of courthouses. They were meant to intimidate." Her voice is low and angry.

I knew about recent campaigns to remove Confederate memorials, but I hadn't connected it to courthouses and the legal system.

"There used to be one in front of the old courthouse here in Hendersonville, but they moved it round back just a few years ago. If you ask me, that statue ought to be moved to a museum or a graveyard somewhere."

"So not leaving a will was intentional?" I ask, trying to understand. I would have guessed it was an oversight, but she is saying something else entirely.

"We took care of our own affairs, Veronica. But it was death either way, wasn't it."

I try to understand what she's saying. "So you lost the land because there was no will. Because you didn't have clear title."

"Something like that," she says. "When there are a lot of heirs, greedy developers like the Thomas family can just come along and manipulate the laws. They took our land twenty years ago. And now they're trying to move me off it."

She pauses and moves slowly as she takes a sip of water from the orange plastic cup sitting on her bed tray, as if telling this story is weakening her. Now that I know she's sick, really sick, I can see her frailty. I can't believe I missed it before. I move the tray closer so she doesn't have to reach as far. I don't understand everything she's saying, but I don't want to upset her further.

"That young man you met is one of the old man's sons."

"Al?" So the man on the ATV, the one I met, is the one evicting my grandmother. He'd been acting nice and neighborly when all along he was the snake my grandmother called him.

"He and his brother want me gone."

"Why all of this now? How long has this been going on?"

"They've been trying to push me out of my house for years, but they served official notice in April."

"They served you written notice in April, Mother Rita? Why are you just now telling me this?" This is not good.

"I tried to fight it on my own. Then I remembered you sell real estate. I figured you could help. I told you it's why I called you down here."

So this is why she called me down here so suddenly. When she'd first mentioned my real estate experience, I hadn't understood how I could help. But these are more recent developments. Maybe there is something I can do, though I'm not sure what.

"Mother Rita, I'm not a lawyer," I say slowly. I don't even half understand this heirs' property she's talking about.

"I have a court date in two weeks." She turns her head and looks over at me. "I know you're leaving soon. Will you come back for it?"

She looks so exhausted that I don't know whether to take her by the hand or call for the nurse. I can't believe she has been trying to fight this battle alone. Having friends and community is one thing. Having blood family is another. And she is mine.

"Of course I will." I try to remember the balance in my savings account. I'm going to have to tell Mama everything. I have no choice. "I'm really sorry all this is happening. We'll find a way out of this. I promise."

She squeezes my hand, and for a second, I see a flash of strength in her eyes.

PART
TWO

EIGHTEEN

Luella

Working together, the women made use of the seasons. In late fall, after the first frost, we began the work of pickling and preserving for winter. In spring, we gathered herbs and filled the jars embossed with "HAPPY LAND LINIMENT." In summer we harvested flowers, fruits, and vegetables and sold them by the roadside. All year long, we delivered liniment to people's houses, places of work, and churches, dried and cured meat after a fresh kill, took in sewing and mending. Before long, our contributions to the kingdom treasury was mighty.

On one of them cold winter afternoons in early 1877, just a year after Robert moved into the palace with me, when the weather was so bad that the three of us had to huddle around the fire as we tried to go about our work, Jola stood in the middle of the room just staring at me.

"What you looking at?"

"I'm looking at you."

"Why you looking at me? Something stained my dress?" I looked down.

"The only thing about to stain your dress is milk."

"What? Girl, stop talking crazy—" I clasped a hand to my mouth. Could she be right? My body had felt different lately, but I'd been so busy I'd ignored it. I'd never been pregnant, so I hadn't recognized the early signs. But right away, I knew Jola was right.

I couldn't speak. For so long, I hadn't thought I was able.

Jola wrapped her arms around me. "Finally. Our dear queen Luella is going be a mama."

I started to cry. "I got to tell Robert."

"Shhh. Just take a minute. Once you share it with him the whole kingdom'll know."

Jola was right. There was no rush to tell. I touched my belly.

"I got to get home," Rachel said abruptly, pulling her shawl up around her shoulders. She tried to brush past me, but I grabbed her and planted a kiss on her cheek. There was a lot of ways to be queen that didn't involve wearing a crown of flowers.

"You going make a good mama, Luella. I truly am happy for you," she said. "It's just my own babies come back to me all of the sudden." I gave her another squeeze.

After she left, a smile managed to escape my lips. A baby! I didn't think I'd ever been happier, not even the day I promised myself to Robert.

ROBERT WASN'T THE kind of man who insisted I sit down just because I was pregnant. If the baby wanted me to sit down, he said I should sit. If the baby said keep going, keep going. But at night he fed me straight from a spoon. And I loved every minute of his attention. My mama had died giving birth to me, and Robert knew I worried about that. So he did what he could to make me believe both me and this baby would be just fine.

In slavery times, we had been worked so hard, a family could barely celebrate a new baby. It was one of the first things we women loved about freedom. We could cherish our bodies, especially during the times when we was busy with the special work of creating life.

I knew it with the eye of a seer that this baby would be a girl-child who would look like my mama. I was looking forward to when I would have time to spend with my daughter, nestle her to my breast, talk to her about good things. I wanted her to learn from the women in the kingdom, be raised by all of us. How to sew. How to cook. How to make the liniment. How to plant a garden. How to do her hair. I wanted her to be useful and a helpmeet to her husband if she married. And if she didn't marry, if she wanted to do something else, that would be hers to decide. Maybe she would be the one to build a house or chop firewood. Maybe she would move up North and preach for women's rights. Just the thought of my daughter speaking her mind made my breath catch in my throat.

Not long after we discovered we was growing our family, Robert took extra work with a nearby white shoemaker. All this time we had bought our shoes from the man, but the shoemaker, who was without children or a wife, was ill and had decided he would leave his shop tools to the kingdom and teach us his trade before passing on to the next life.

We offered one of our young boys, but the man would only trust his knowledge with Robert, the king. So Robert began to walk the three miles or so to the man's shop, where he would begin

157

the early morning by cutting leather. Robert enjoyed the work and came home each evening excited to talk about what new skill he'd learned that day. The shoemaker was a kind and patient teacher, and he'd earned Robert's respect. I was sure that Robert was an excellent student; smart as he was, the man could learn anything.

Robert returned to the kingdom later and later, until he was returning after the dinner hour and I had to keep his food warm in the hearth. One night, while I was waiting, somebody started pounding the drum. It sounded like music, but I knew it was an alarm. I stepped out on the porch, worried. The drum wasn't used much these days. Robert often came home late, but surely this didn't have nothing to do with him. I placed a hand on top of my belly.

I could make out three men walking up the lane. As they neared, I saw that it was two men on either side of Robert, propping him up.

"What happened?" I nearly jumped off the porch. Robert's eye was swollen, his shirt torn.

"Get him in the house," yelled Hal.

We brought him inside and placed him carefully in the chair. I sent one of the women to fill a bowl with water, and when she came back, I moistened a cloth and pressed it to his eye.

Nobody said much because we all knew this kind of violence. We just focused on making him comfortable. It was not a time for talking because rage was not far behind words.

THE COUNCIL USUALLY met every full moon when the light was brightest, but this meeting was called halfway through the cycle. I sat on the council now along with Margaret, Reverend Couch's wife. She'd earned the second seat as the eldest woman in the kingdom. Without a doubt, the woman knew things. Some even said she was the one who directed her husband's missions in search of new residents. During meetings, she sat quietly and listened, not offering an opinion unless asked.

On the other hand, I was the bold one. At times, the men regarded Margaret with a pleading look, as if to ask that she shut me up. But she never did.

"Forgive me, brothers, for disrupting your evening," began Robert. I tried to signal to him, but he didn't look my way. He usually addressed me and Margaret, too, but he had neglected to do that tonight. It had been two weeks since he'd been beaten, and he still hadn't told me what happened that night. My husband was still hurting on the inside.

It was spring, but chilly. We was all wrapped in blankets and sitting close. The other men on the council—Sam, John Earl, Hal, Harry, Thomas, George, and Papa—regarded Robert solemnly. It seemed Robert was finally ready to talk about what happened. I just wished he'd spoken to me first. By not telling me, he hadn't allowed me to be a queen, and I needed to be that for him and for the kingdom.

"As y'all know, I met a bit of trouble on my way back home from the shoemaker's shop recently. I done had another visit on that same road."

Another visit? So that made it two things he hadn't shared. I turned my face to hide my hurt.

"They want money," he continued.

"Who want money?" Papa demanded.

"The law. They say we got to pay them if we want to be safe. Otherwise, they can't be responsible if some lowlifes was to attack us again."

"Lowlifes," Papa repeated.

"They say the men that attacked me don't like us up here on this hill. Say they can protect us if we pay."

"The men."

I could hear it in his voice. Papa had enough experience with the Klan to know that these *lowlifes, men,* and *the law* was likely all the same.

"Robert, this land belong to the Widow Davis. Sound like they got business with her," George added.

"They already talked to her and her son. They ain't paying," Robert said.

"But we been here for four years now," said John Earl. "Why they just now messing with us?"

"Maybe that's why. The longer we here and show what we can do on our own, the more they want to take it away. I reckon they heard Mr. Horne giving us his shoe shop and they don't want to buy shoes from us." Robert shrugged, as if he was too tired to sort it all out.

"But your brother said if we didn't vote, they'd leave us be," John Earl pressed him.

"Voting ain't the only thing that get in their craw," said Hal.

George reached a hand out from under his blanket and stroked his beard. "If we don't pay, what they going do?"

You remember what the Klan was like back home. Wasn't no strangers on them horses.

So you saying they want us to pay them to protect us from them?

They think we living up here off the fat of the land and they want a piece.

A piece of what? We don't even own this land.

They know we working the railroad. They probably know we got money stored up.

Somebody been flapping they lips.

How much they asking for?

Two dollars a month.

Two dollars a month? To hell with the law.

Robert waited patiently until the chatter died down. "I say we pay it. Get them off our backs for now."

My insides churned, and it wasn't because of the baby. I had a feeling this wouldn't be the last of their demands. If the Widow wouldn't protect us from them, then we was at their mercy. Today it would be two dollars, tomorrow it would be four. I looked at Margaret and could tell from the look on her face she was thinking the same.

"It's time we go to the Widow and ask to buy some land. We been good to her family."

"You think owning this land will keep us from having to pay more than that one day?" Hal asked.

"I think the only thing white men respect is property. If we own this land, then they accept us as citizens. No choice but to. Then they can't come over here trying to scare us because we landowners."

I wanted to believe Robert. All of us did.

I DELIVERED CORDELIA on Christmas Day in 1877. She was born with a head full of hair and a birthmark in the shape of a fish on her leg. Nobody doted on her more than Robert. As soon as she was old enough to hold her head up, she would finish drinking from my breast and he would tie her into a cloth on his back just as women did.

Cordelia delighted in her daddy and rarely cried when he took her, giving me time to finish my work. After Cordelia had soiled her cloth and the stink was intolerable, he'd bring her to me and stand back, patiently waiting while I cleaned her up and fed her. Then he would wrap her up until only her eyes peeked out before fixing her to his back again. I didn't think he'd known how big his heart could grow. Robert had said he didn't need children, but he sure did act like he'd been praying for her all his life.

I truly believe he got over the humiliation of that beating by looking into his baby's face each morning.

Robert was still working with the shoemaker, who had somehow escaped death's call but still kept up with his end of the promise. Now Robert returned before nightfall, rushing to be with us for dinner. He praised every little step the baby took, as if she was the first baby in the world to smile or grow a tooth. Even my papa listened to Robert's boasting patiently, letting him go on and on in his love-drunk state. The baby brought my husband back to me, filled him with a joy no lowlife could kill.

At times, I wondered if the news had reached William that his brother and me had been blessed in this way, but I dared not bring it up lest I break the spell. As soon as the promise of summer began to warm the air, Cordelia demanded to be outside. If I brought her in the house she would cry, but as soon as I took her outside and sat on the porch she would settle. She loved being out in the sun and would turn her face up to it so often that we had to oil her down to protect her. People would remark on it: *That baby sure do love the sun.*

Soon Robert took to calling her "Sunny," and the name stuck.

NINETEEN

Nikki

For Mother Rita's dinner, I made macaroni and cheese, baked sweet potatoes, and roasted broccoli. Everything turned out better than I'd hoped. I made too much food for just me and Mother Rita, so I invite Maddie Mae over to eat the rest of it with me that night. I make up the table in the back room so we can enjoy the cool.

"I brought pie." Maddie Mae holds up a foil-covered dish. "I already had a slice, but I didn't know I was coming until half an hour ago."

I take the dish from her. "Sorry for the last-minute invitation."

"You disturbed my movie."

"Hopefully it was one you've seen before. You made this pie?"

"No, my chef made it."

I giggle. These mountain women have a sense of humor, and I'm starting to dig it.

"I owe you an apology, too," she says. "I'm sorry for the way I broke the news to you the other day. That wasn't very neighborly of me." She's wearing a blue and white caftan that drapes on her body like an evening gown. Her gray hair is picked out in a soft afro.

"You don't need to apologize. I'm glad somebody around here was honest with me for a change."

"Rita wasn't happy with me."

I open the refrigerator door. Mother Rita drank all the wine; otherwise, I'd pour Maddie Mae a glass.

The track and field championships are on television, and Maddie Mae settles at the table, as if she's done it a thousand times before in that exact chair. She probably has, considering how close she and Mother Rita are. No wonder Maddie Mae keeps dipping in our business. She's as close to a nosy great-auntie as I'll ever get. I go back to the kitchen for the serving dishes, setting the food on the table as it comes out of the oven.

"Miss Maddie?"

She tsks. "I told you about that Miss."

"Do you want me to get you something else before I sit down?"

"I know where the kitchen is." Her voice is kind but firm. I try not to compare her to Mother Rita, but it's nearly impossible. A breeze drifts through the screen, and I welcome the relief of this simple dinner with her.

Mother Rita's spirits were good when I visited her that afternoon. The doctors said they were planning her discharge for tomorrow morning. She was wearing a clean gown, and the blanket I'd found on the shelf of her bedroom closet was folded neatly across her feet. I'd also taken her a vase of zinnias. She had inspected them and complimented me on my cutting.

"Mother Rita comes home tomorrow," I tell Maddie Mae.

She spoons some macaroni on her plate. "I know she's happy about that."

"I'm still planning to leave on Sunday. You and Bryan have my phone number. Y'all call me if you need me."

She grunts.

I can tell she disapproves of this decision, but I don't have the ability to solve all these problems in one day. My grandmother called me down here because she thinks I'm some knowledgeable property expert when, in fact, I'm not even a licensed broker. I'm just an agent. If Mother Rita can't figure it out with all her book smarts, I'm not sure what makes her think I can do it. "You know, I think it might be impossible for Mother Rita to get this land back if it's already sold."

"Hmm." She wrinkles her forehead.

"I'll be back for the court date. But look, I'm not a miracle worker."

"Child, do you even have any faith?" She stabs the macaroni with her fork.

After a few minutes of eating, I say, "You know, I can understand Mother Rita and Mama had their issues with each other. But why drag me into it?"

The gun goes off, and a race erupts on the television. The runners take off, but the camera focuses on a woman whose ponytail flows behind her as she pulls ahead of the rest. Her hands fan out beside her, pumping. A smile teases the edges of her lips, as if the running is easy.

Maddie Mae puts down her fork and gets up from her chair. She leaves the room, and when she returns, she's carrying a wooden box.

She places the box in front of me and I stare at it. It's an ordinary box, worn at the corners, the kind easily found at a craft store. "What's this?"

"Open it."

I can't move. I don't know what's inside, but I know it's going to hit me with a force I am not prepared for. *This is why you came to Hendersonville, Nikki. This is the reason.*

"Open it." She begins to eat her food again.

On television, the athlete is crying. She has won the race and wears a flag draped across her back. They appear to be tears of joy, but it's hard to tell. That kind of joy always carries a tinge of relief.

Before I can open the box, I have to ask her something, because Mother Rita refuses to be straight with me about her health, as with so many other things. "My grandmother says the doctors told her she only has months to live. Is that true?"

"She's dying, Nikki. It's not easy for me to say that out loud, but it's the truth. And you being here"—she pauses—"is a blessing for her."

"She asked me to come."

"She wants you to help get the land back. But that's not the only reason. I believe she wants to make peace with her family."

I place a hand on top of the box. There's no latch. It's a simple rectangular box, about twelve inches wide.

"So why didn't she call Mama instead of me?" My voice drifts.

"Family is complicated, Nikki. You and I aren't going to solve all the problems of the Lovejoy family in one day."

I wonder if Mama would even want to come. Every time I mention Mother Rita's name, she shuts down. That damage could be irreparable in this lifetime. I understand that. But it doesn't mean it isn't sad. I am a casualty of their war. Me and now Shawnie.

I use a fingernail to push up the lid. Inside there are pieces of folded white paper. I pick up one of them and unfold it. It's a photocopy of Mama's ninth-grade report card. I open another one.

"Those are your mother's report cards from high school. Did you know she was a straight A student?"

I hadn't assumed my mother was a poor student; I just hadn't known she was an excellent student because no one ever told me.

"They wrote her up in the paper for it. Rita and Herbert were so proud." She watches me as I sift through the papers. "She kept yours, too."

"My what?"

"High school report cards. Your mother sent them to her."

I look up at her, startled. Those were the days when the two women were speaking. I think back to the day Mama told me Mother Rita was no longer in *our* lives.

Beneath the stack of Mama's report cards is a schedule of my soccer team from nearly thirty years ago. A photo of the trophy we won. My eighth-grade graduation program. Copies of my high school newspaper naming honor roll students with my name underlined. My high school graduation program. And an original letter of my acceptance to Howard, the university we ultimately couldn't afford. I haven't seen any of this stuff in years. Envelopes bear Mama's handwriting with Mother Rita's address written out neatly, but there are no personal letters from her. It's as if she stuffed these mementos into the mail with no accompanying note of affection. Even with the chilly winds between them, Mother Rita greedily saved all of it, a proud grandmother cherishing her granddaughter's life.

"Mother Rita was an only child," Maddie says. "She and Herbert hadn't been married five years before she lost both her mother and father, within a year of each other. So Herbert and your mother were her world. Then you came along, and you were her world, too."

I am speechless. The love in this box is indisputable.

"Do you see who you are now? You've always been special to her."

I press the box to my chest. It is as if there are a thousand arms wrapped around me.

"Rita and I grew up together. We always planned to see after each other in our old age. But I had a grandson to help me if she left before I did. I always wished for her to have family, too, in case my number came up first. Now that you're here, I'm hoping we can all be there for her. It's time for y'all Lovejoys to get your act together and cherish the days you got left."

"I don't know how." My grandmother has loved me ever since I was born. Now she's dying and the moments have passed.

She comes behind me and turns me around by the shoulders. I feel dizzy, but her touch steadies me. "What's outside that window?" she asks.

"I can't see anything. It's pitch-black dark."

"Sometimes what you can't see is right there in front of you. But you got to look, look! This right here is the prettiest land you ever set eyes on. And your family has fought for generations to hold on to it. For you, Nikki. They wanted it for your mama and for you and for Shawnie. This ain't just some old-time legend. This is yours," Maddie says.

My food has grown cold on my plate.

"What I'm trying to tell you," Maddie Mae continues, "is that you can't leave on Sunday. I know you have things to get back to, and maybe you've got to handle those things. But I'm urging you, begging you, to stay a little while longer. Don't walk out on your legacy and birthright."

Like my mama did? I want to say. Maddie Mae doesn't appear to leave her sentence unfinished, but I can't help myself.

TWENTY

Luella

By 1878, the kingdom had grown to over a hundred people, and the Saluda Grade railroad was completed with the help of men from the kingdom alongside convicts from the state prison. Men died building the railroad, especially along the steepest parts. Fortunately, we didn't lose none of the kingdom men. Its completion meant business at the inn slowed as trains went right on past it before passengers stopped for lodging. A trip that used to take two weeks by coach from the Carolina coast now took two days by rail. It also meant our men didn't have as much work hauling up and down the turnpike.

The importance of the women's work grew. With the use of ginseng and sassafras, the liniment was selling fast. More than fast. We could barely keep up with the sales. Now we grew most of our own food, and there was plenty of game in the woods to hunt and eat. But we still needed supplies the kingdom couldn't provide. When we'd first arrived, we'd bartered. The women would walk up and down the turnpike with a cart, and when travelers approached we'd wave them down, trading all sorts of things—flint or flower oils or even baskets we'd woven—for whatever we needed—salt, sugar, coffee. We didn't have much when we arrived, having sold most everything back in South Carolina, but we had made our way over the past five years.

Nearly all of the kingdom men worked in the zircon mines in Webster County at least some of the time. Occasionally, they brought back reports about William. I asked if he'd taken another wife and family, but they said no. He knew about my marriage to Robert and the birth of our Sunny, and he sent us a blessing. I felt the sting of that blessing even as I craved it. I just didn't understand why he kept passing along messages instead of coming in the flesh to talk to me.

One day, Robert came back to the cabin carrying Sunny and set her on my lap. She was just starting to walk, and he liked to take her out so she could walk in the soft grass. She was hungry and fussy, so I put her right to my breast.

"We got enough," he said.

"Enough what?" At first, I thought he was talking about our little family. Now that we knew we could make them, surely he didn't mean enough children.

"We got enough money to buy land from the Widow."

I could barely allow myself to believe it. I knew how much William had wanted this, how hard all of us in this community had worked to own a piece of this hill. The years of sweat. The nights imagining what such a purchase could mean for us. "How much we got?"

"Enough."

"You taking it to the council this week?" I asked.

"Sure enough. We got to have a vote."

A vote. What was there to vote about? Yes, yes, yes to all the land we could hold. Nobody could object to that. In my excitement, I couldn't help but feel honored that Robert was telling me before taking it to the council.

"And how much land you plan on asking about?"

"I don't know. But if the council say yes, I'd like you to go with me to the inn. The Widow might look upon us more favorable if you and me go together. If she agree, I'm figuring we put half the land in your name and the other half in mines."

"My name?" The suggestion shocked me so I almost dropped Sunny. I wrapped my arms around her thick waist.

"Now, woman, why you repeating after me? Your ears working?" He laughed, but I was still looking sideways at him.

I knew what he was thinking. We didn't have a marriage paper, and that might be a good thing in the eyes of the law. We could protect each piece if somebody came after us. A surge of pride rose in my chest. A colored woman landowner!

"You think the Widow might be more inclined to agree if she think a husband and wife taking care of the property?" I tried to slow my heartbeat.

"People in this country got a fixation with land. Even when they need to sell it, it's got a piece of them. She need to feel something when we go up there. Like it'll be in good hands."

I rarely visited the inn these days, and since business had slowed after the railroad was finished, we was expecting the Widow to ask for rent on the land soon. We needed to go now.

"I want you to put on a nice dress, but don't do yourself up too much. Remember we want that white woman to help us."

I understood. In order to convince them to help us, they had to first feel sorry for us. But we also had to look respectable. It was an impossible knot to tie.

"Alright, I'll talk to Margaret. When the council meets, we'll be ready." Sunny was done eating and had dozed off.

He kissed me on the forehead, then Sunny, and walked back outside to finish his work.

THE DAY WE was to meet with the Widow, I rose early to wash my hair in the creek. One thing was for sure, I did not want to stink up that white woman's parlor. My hair had grown longer during my pregnancy, and even the comb Robert gave me couldn't untangle it completely. At the creek, I unfurled my braid, then dipped my head to the side so the hair could soak. I rubbed a bar of soap through it and rinsed until the water ran clear. I weaved my hair back into a braid and tucked it into a bun. Papa had never wanted me to cut my hair, always saying it reminded him of Mama. But at the end of the next winter, I would finally cut it. I was a mother now and caring for Sunny's hair was more than enough.

I chose an unstained dress in a dull brown color. Jola had let it out after the baby was born so I could still fit. It didn't have the buttons to allow me to nurse, so I fed Sunny before I put the dress on. After Sunny ate, she sat up watching me, quiet, as if she knew I was going somewhere important.

By the time Robert arrived back at the cabin with Jola, I was ready.

"Don't worry about this baby none, I got her," Jola said. "If she get hungry I'll take her over to Penny's cabin. She still nursing her baby and can feed Sunny, too."

"Tell her she trying to walk so keep an eye out."

"Woman, you ain't the first to birth a baby." Jola smiled and pulled me into a hug. She still hadn't married, and I knew she had no mind for it. "Make sure you smile. Your smile can soften that old widow's heart."

Robert looked at me as she said this, as if he was seeing me through Jola's eyes. Admiration glistened on his face, and I blushed beneath his gaze.

"Y'all going or y'all standing around making eyes at each other all day," said Jola.

Robert took my hand. "Come on, Queen. Time for us to go buy our people a kingdom."

We took the back path through the woods, the same path the men traveled when moving between the kingdom and the turnpike, the way the women took when they went to the inn in the morning and returned to the kingdom at night.

We walked quickly because we wanted to arrive early and wait for the Widow rather than have her waiting on us. Robert was excited, walking so fast I struggled to match his long strides in my dress. Every now and then he turned back and took my arm to help me over a puddle or a fallen branch. Then he walked ahead of me again.

At that hour, all was quiet. We crossed the turnpike and walked up the hill to the house built by the Widow's late father-in-law. Eventually, the family had turned it into an inn when they hit hard times before the war. At the height of their wealth, the Davises owned a thousand acres and the humans to till it. When the war came, all their people left. Some moved to Flat Rock while others wandered off to find family, never to return to this part of North Carolina again. When the old man died during the war, the Widow struggled. Robert and William had met the Davises during their time traveling up and down the turnpike working on behalf of J. D. Montgomery. But it was William the Davises trusted. Robert was the younger brother who sat back while his older brother did the talking. We didn't know how they'd think of Robert now, even if he was the king and our leader.

We approached the back of the house where the back door opened to the kitchen. Though Hester the cook was busy with breakfast preparations, she supplied us a damp rag. Me and Robert sat on the back porch steps, wiping off the bits of mud and dirt that had stuck to our shoes. Hester knew the purpose of our visit. Word had quietly passed through the kingdom, and everybody was waiting anxiously for the outcome.

The cook led us to a room where early arrivals was usually asked to wait for their accommodations to be readied. The house smelled of bacon fat, and though me and Robert had been served a large breakfast that morning in preparation for our visit, neither of us had been able to eat much. I hoped my stomach wouldn't start talking.

Chairs crowded the small space, arranged in no particular order. It was a room for waiting, not entertaining. There was a low table where the guest might be served a refreshment and a small shelf crammed with books they might read while waiting. The corner of the room was bare, a place for trunks to be placed before being carried upstairs.

Robert, straight-backed in his jacket, sat still, a wall of calm. I took his hand in mine and squeezed his fingers. He managed a small cough.

After a long wait, the Widow and her son entered the room.

These days, she was even thinner, with a gaunt face and hollows beneath her eyes. Even in the times of prosperity following our arrival, she had never lost the look of grief. I couldn't remember if I'd ever seen the woman smile. There was an air of resignation about her, about her circumstance, as a woman facing the future alone. Her son was the man of the house, but he was generally an indolent fellow and not seemingly very interested in the affairs of the inn. When he did insert himself, it was ill-timed. He fancied himself a poet, which the Widow did not appear to regard with seriousness. It was impossible to know whether he was good at it, given her disregard.

The son walked ahead of his mother, exchanging pleasantries and asking us to please return to our seats. He had been educated in the North and had picked up certain mannerisms. He didn't have the coarseness of some of the white men we had known in South Carolina. He crossed one leg over the other while seated and had a habit of waving his right hand in the air when speaking. He shook Robert's hand and smiled, though no one offered us refreshments. We had served in these houses long enough to know that this lack of courtesy was a slight.

The Widow curtly nodded as greeting. Her son asked about our business and Robert began.

"We been here living on the property for over four years now. We been working here in the inn, faithfully serving your family. We been loyal . . ."—he searched for the right word—". . . workers. And we hoping y'all agree."

"Yes, that is true," the son responded, "you have been loyal"— and here he also searched for the right word—"people. And we have paid you for that, have we not?"

"Yes, you paid us fairly. And you treated us real fair. We sure appreciate that."

We had not been paid in money, had only been allowed to live on the land. Though the arrangement was not without value, we understood that even though we wasn't paid the same as white people for the same work, we was expected to be grateful. This was a leap from our previous circumstance, and we could never express enough gratitude. There just wasn't enough thank-yous to satisfy.

"We come this morning to ask about the land," said Robert.

We never used the word *kingdom* with the Davis family. Without a doubt, they knew we called it a kingdom and claimed the titles of king and queen, though they probably thought it was the folly of Negroes.

"We would like to buy a little bit of your land. There's so much of it. We understand this is good land, and we want to know if you might be willing to part with a piece."

I glanced at him. Robert was nervous, but there was no other way to ask other than outright.

"You mean pay us for it?" the Widow asked, speaking for the first time.

"Yes, ma'am," I interrupted. "Our men been working the railroad all these years, and you know we been selling our liniment. I brought you some."

I passed her a jar, and she unscrewed the cap, sniffing it. The scent of sassafras brought a smile to her lips. I smiled back, remembering what Jola had told me about softening her up.

"I've been using it. I like it very much even though I'm sorry we couldn't sell it in the inn. This was your idea, Luella?"

"Yes, Missus."

"I ain't trading this land for liniment," said her son.

"You have money?" the Widow asked, screwing the cap back on and sliding the jar into the pocket of her dress.

"Yes, Missus," Robert said. "We want to pay you with money. Real money."

"How much land are we talking about?" The Widow's interest was undeniable. Sweat beaded on her upper lip. Watching her, I could see that she was more than willing to sell, though whether we could agree on a price was a different matter.

"We'd like to buy enough for our people."

"How many acres, William?"

She'd called him by his brother's name. Robert didn't flinch at the mistake. One of the men on the council had suggested we ask to purchase a hundred acres.

"We'd like to purchase two hundred acres," Robert responded.

I held my breath. I didn't know how many acres the Davises owned these days. Was we asking for too much? Would we be able to afford it? Robert was good with numbers, but he wasn't his brother.

"Mother, we ought to charge rent, not sell—"

The Widow held up a hand to silence her son, then tapped her walking cane once on the floor. Hester appeared in the doorway. The Widow had given the signal to end our little meeting.

"We would like to consider your offer and determine a fair price. When we have a number, we will send for you."

We stood, and the son did not respond to Robert's extended hand so my husband dropped his arm to his side. The Widow watched me, and I couldn't tell what she was thinking, but if I had to guess, I would say she was watching me with new eyes.

Two weeks later, the Davises called us back to the inn. For two hundred dollars in full, they offered 75 acres on the South Carolina side of the mountain and 130 acres on the North Carolina side, a little over the amount we'd asked for. I knew without a doubt, Widow Davis had been the one to make this happen.

Though it was bought with our communal treasury, the deed had to be in a name. The council agreed to deed the South Carolina portion to Robert and the North Carolina portion to me. The women in the kingdom was real happy with this arrangement. Land in a woman's name was cause for celebration. That night, the drumhead echoed throughout the kingdom.

TWENTY-ONE

Nikki

The next morning is Friday, and I'm supposed to go home in two days. When I'd called Bryan the night before, he'd already known about the eviction and promised to make a few calls. Now I call him back three times before he finally answers.

"I found a lawyer who might be able to help," he says. "She's an estate planning lawyer. Want to drive to Asheville with me?"

"Can we go today?"

"I got the day off. I can be there within the hour."

The trip from Hendersonville to Asheville is only about twenty miles, but the interstate is tricky. There's construction, which narrows the traffic into two lanes and means the tractor trailers cruise right alongside us, too close for my comfort, though it doesn't seem to faze Bryan. He drives a late-model Nissan Altima, and it's immaculately clean, the type of clean that only a single man can maintain. It was impossible for me to keep a clean car when Shawnie was a child, though now that she's older, I still keep a messy car. It didn't help that as soon as she got her driver's license, she treated my car no better than she treated her bedroom.

Bryan isn't a fast driver. That gives us plenty of time to chat.

"So your daughter graduated high school? Is she planning to go to college?"

"She wants to take some classes at University of the District of Columbia, but she plans to work full-time."

"What does she want to study?"

"She's not sure yet." I don't feel like talking about Shawnie at the moment. Mother Rita's hearing date is on my mind, and I'm really hoping this lawyer can help us.

"I bet you sell a lot of houses. My buddy left D.C. because it was too expensive to buy a house there."

"Yes, that's true." I look out the window.

"How did you get into real estate?"

"What?"

"I said, how did you get into selling houses?"

How did I get into this career? I followed Darius. Took advantage of the housing market boom that happened twenty years ago. Couldn't figure out what else to do. There are a lot of ways I can answer that question. It's all so fuzzy now. Instead, I say vaguely, "I don't really remember."

He glances at me. "Hey, the lawyer will know what to do. Mother Rita won't have to move."

I'm grateful for his help, and I really should be kinder to him.

"I'm sorry. I'm not a great conversationalist today."

"I understand," he says.

I see genuine care lines in his forehead. Maybe light conversation is what we both need. "What about you? What's your story?"

"Let's see. I went to UNC Asheville. Majored in English. Got my master's in library science."

"No kids?"

"I dated somebody for a long time. She had two sons from a previous relationship. They're in high school now. Even though I don't date their mother anymore, I still go to all their games. The older one is a three-star recruit. I'm proud of him."

I turn my head toward him. Bryan isn't a bad-looking guy. Well-groomed with impeccable manners. I can't imagine how the women in this town are allowing him to sit around single. Or maybe he isn't single. I'm too shy to ask.

"I've been meaning to thank you for being such a friend to my grandmother. You're more than just her librarian."

"My mom passed away when I was in college. Mrs. Lovejoy is like a mother and grandmother to me all wrapped up in one."

"I'm sorry about your mom."

"Thanks."

"I lost my dad eight years ago."

He takes his eyes off the road and looks over at me for a full second. "I didn't know that."

"Mother Rita came for the funeral. That was the last time I saw her."

His eyes are back on the road. "Maybe that's why you looked so sad when I first saw you. Are you glad to have your grandmother back in your life?"

I don't know how much he knows about my family rift. I'm surprised he thinks I looked sad when I arrived. I had a lot of emotions swirling around inside, but sadness? That wasn't how I'd put it. Still, he noticed something. I'm trying to figure out how to answer the question when my phone buzzes in my lap and I let it go to voicemail. A moment later, a text appears on the screen.

Nikki, I hope you're keeping in better touch with Shawnie than you are with me, your own mother. What kind of work conference are you at?

I turn the phone face down. "I think you might be the first Black male librarian I've ever met."

"You need to get to the public library more."

"Touché. But come on, it can't be that common."

He smiles. "I'm just playing with you. You're right. There need to be more of us. I decided to become a librarian when a professor in college suggested it. Nobody had ever mentioned it to me. I thought it sounded like a good life. Hey, I get to be around books all day and meet interesting people."

As we get closer to Asheville, the interstate widens, and he expertly guides the car toward the exit.

"So what kinds of questions are we going to be asking this lawyer?" I ask.

"There's only one question: How can we stop the eviction?"

"I'm still trying to understand everything that happened with this heirs' property situation."

"If there's any chance of getting the land back, R.J. can help us," he says.

"That's his name?"

"R. J. Parker." He nods. "And she's a she."

Nervously, I begin to think I'm in over my head. I don't know the first thing about how much this will cost. I wonder if Mother

Rita has a nest egg. We made a little over four hundred dollars selling flowers on Thursday, though I'm not sure how many weddings she has booked this summer. According to Bryan, this R. J. Parker is meeting with us today as a personal favor, but in order to move forward we will inevitably need money. I have a retirement account through my brokerage, but as a single woman I maintain a strict rule not to touch it.

"Alright, this is it." Bryan parks the car right next to the handicap space and unbuckles his seat belt. "I've met R.J. before. She's good people. You'll like her."

As soon as we walk into R.J.'s office, I understand what Bryan meant. R.J. has big, curly hair and wears bright red lipstick. She has a Diana Ross kind of glamour, and I like her instantly.

"Hey, Bryan, how you doing, sweetie?" She comes from behind her desk.

"Alright, alright. This is Nikki, Mrs. Lovejoy's granddaughter. They're the family that live on the kingdom land."

"Ah, yes, the kingdom land. Come on in, y'all. I already got John making us some lemonade. He'll bring it in a second."

Something about this R.J. makes me immediately trust her. I wonder if that's her talent, how she can move a judge. She fills the little office with her presence.

"Miss Nikki, where you from?"

"D.C."

"Oh, okay. You spent much time down here?"

I shake my head.

"I see. You should know the kingdom is a local legend around here. I grew up hearing about it. There's a lot of rumors, of course. And a lot of misinformation and lies, I'm sure." She laughs. "But I grew up hearing about it."

"Oh, really? What'd you hear?" It's still odd to me that my mama never mentioned it.

"I actually had family who lived on the land. The Caseys. My great-great-grandfather was a Casey. Actually, maybe that's three greats. Or four. I can't keep up."

"I didn't know you had history with the kingdom," Bryan interrupts.

"Sure did. That's why I agreed to the meeting."

"So your family must've known mine," I say.

"I don't see how they couldn't. They say your ancestor was the queen. Of course, I only half believe some of those old stories."

"You don't think there was a king and queen?"

She tilts her head. "To tell you the truth, I don't know what to believe. I know they came up here after slavery and made a home on the mountain. And I've heard tales about a king and a queen, but a lot of it comes from some 1950s pamphlet."

"Patton," I say. "She interviewed a few of the descendants."

"And I'm sure she embellished."

"Sounds likely. But my grandmother says our account of the kingdom came directly down to us through the women in the family. Patton corroborates at least some of those oral stories."

"You sound like a believer," she says.

I consider that. Am I? "Well, we know they lived there. The only thing that's in question is the story of the kingdom and the royal titles. That's the part that seems far-fetched."

"I was always impressed that they were landowners," R.J. says. "That couldn't have been easy."

"My grandmother says her mother inherited nearly fifty acres that she passed down. Mother Rita lost the land due to heirs' property, something about some distant cousin." I shrug, but R.J. doesn't crack a smile.

"Unfortunately, land loss due to heirs' property is common." R.J. turns to her computer and types quickly with her impossibly long nails.

"I don't really understand it," I say.

She turns back to me. "When someone dies without a will, the heirs become tenants-in-common. Depending on the family, sometimes there are a lot of heirs. And each one of them has the right to transfer their individual share of land."

"You mean they can sell their share without the other heirs' permission?" Bryan asks.

"Correct. Some greedy developer comes in, buys the share of some unsuspecting relative for a paltry amount because this distant relative has no connection to the land whatsoever even though he's a rightful heir. The developer then goes to a judge and forces a sale of the entire property. The land goes up for auction, but the other heirs aren't properly notified that the land is being auctioned on the courthouse steps, so to speak—"

"And it sells for far less than market value," I finish.

"Bingo."

"And this forced sale is legal?" My grandmother woke up one day and the land had literally been sold out from under her feet.

"Nikki, we have lost millions of acres to heirs' property law. I haven't done a lot of these cases, but a friend of mine does them down in South Carolina. He says coastal Carolina is ground zero for heirs' property losses."

Of course it is. Coastal property in South Carolina is worth millions in today's market. If there is a way for greedy developers to get that property under market value and move Black families off the land, I'm sure they're taking it.

"Do you have any of this where you are?" she asks. "Bryan tells me you're in real estate."

"I only sell in the city, and I haven't ever faced this issue specifically," I say, thinking aloud. "In D.C., we run a title search to confirm chain of title. When I sell a property, the settlement company usually has a company they contract to run the title search to make sure there aren't any claimants out there who aren't on the deed or there aren't any existing liens on the property. Then the purchaser buys title insurance that most lenders require. But what we're talking about here is something different."

"Yes, a little different." She leans forward. "Black folks lost their land in all kinds of predatory ways. Racial terror. Lynching. Intentionally increased taxes that they couldn't afford. And sometimes outright theft. Some estimate that African Americans lost nearly 90 percent of their land over the course of the twentieth century. A lot of that land loss was due to heirs' property."

"Ninety percent of our land?" I'm astounded by this figure. I look over at Bryan as if for his confirmation that this is true, but he's listening, too. "What does that even mean?"

"Nikki, we're talking about hundreds of billions of dollars in lost land," she says.

"Hundreds of billions? That can't be right."

"That sounds like a major source of the racial wealth gap in this country," Bryan says.

"Major source," R.J. repeats.

"No wonder my grandmother is so aggrieved," I whisper.

"It sounds like your grandmother's case is simple. A distant cousin unknowingly sold her out. Now the family who bought it wants to exercise their right of ownership and move her off the land. If they legally hold title, I'm afraid she may not have a way out of this. Once the land has been sold, it's gone. That's why organizations on the ground are trying to prevent it from happening in the first place by getting families together so they can share information. They bring in family members from all over the country and hold information sessions that double as a family reunion of sorts."

"This is all so unfair. Mother Rita's ancestors worked—I mean, my ancestors worked hard to buy that land. It must be worth hundreds of thousands now," I say.

She shakes her head. "Nikki, if your grandmother owned those fifty acres today, they would be worth millions."

Millions? I had no idea property in this part of western North Carolina could be worth that much. I think of what land ownership could have meant for my family. We could have gotten educated, taken loans out to establish businesses, bought and sold real estate during the boom periods.

"You're saying that we lost our generational wealth," I say.

"Yes, I'm afraid so. And as far as I can tell right now, there really isn't a way to get it back," R.J. says.

But it's more than the monetary value. Losing the kingdom has meant we've lost connection as a family and our knowledge of ancestral legacy. We're no longer stewards of the land. Mama no longer puts her hands in the earth, and neither do any of us descendants. Maybe if we still owned a place for repair and refuge, we wouldn't have crumbled into pieces as a family.

"So why does my grandmother think there's still a chance to get it back?"

"I'm sorry to say it's just wishful thinking. I wish I had better news."

187

I struggle to contain myself. This is devastating news.

"Well, we still have this court date," I say finally.

"Yes, and I'm happy to represent her in court. We can try to buy her more time before the eviction. Ah, here's the lemonade. Ooh, and John, you brought us some of those cookies I like. I wouldn't be a good host, Miss Nikki, if I didn't offer my guests some snacks."

I take a sip of the lemonade and pick up a cookie though my stomach is in no mood for it. I never would have guessed Mother Rita's land was worth a small fortune. I think back to my high school history teacher discussing the broken promise of "forty acres and a mule." I remember learning of racially motivated redlining and the predatory loans that targeted Black borrowers. Even now, homes in the areas east of Rock Creek Park in D.C. are underappraised just because of the zip code. That whole history is sitting in the room with us right now.

After her assistant leaves, R.J. turns serious again. "Let me try to find out some more information about the family that owns it. I'm not sure what they plan to do with the land, but if we tell them Mother Rita is sick, they may have a little sympathy and allow her to stay. You could also write them a letter, and they can put up a historical plaque or something to honor the kingdom. I think that's the best you can hope for."

The cookie hangs between my fingers, untouched. I had figured this was the case, but I also know Mother Rita is not going to accept this answer. And I don't have the heart to tell her.

TWENTY-TWO

The next day, the hospital discharges Mother Rita. My conversations with both Maddie Mae and the lawyer haven't left me, but I'm just trying to put one foot in front of the other for now.

First order of business is to get Mother Rita home.

"The doctor says my blood pressure is down and my red blood cell count is normal. I'm good as new," she says energetically during the car ride. My grandmother is dying, so this optimism rings false in my ears.

When we arrive, the house is quiet. It's still early and Mother Rita says she plans to spend some time in her room reading. I wonder if she plans to read or if she just wants to rest in bed.

"Is there anything you need?"

"Can you fill up my water bottle?"

"Of course."

"With ice, please."

I return to her room with the water bottle and set it on her nightstand. The ice cubes make a jingling noise.

"Thank you, baby." She's sitting on the edge of the bed. I don't know if I should help her or if she wants to be left alone, so I try to busy myself by unpacking her duffel bag.

"You find anything else out?" she asks.

I don't have to ask her to clarify. I know she's talking about the land. I avoid her eyes. "I'm not sure if Bryan told you, but we went and visited a lawyer in Asheville. She wasn't exactly a fountain of good news. Do you have any ideas on how we can fight the Thomas brothers?"

"What's ours is ours. They can't take it away from us."

"I understand what you're saying from a moral standpoint. Really, I do. But the law is different. R.J. says even if Fred Thomas took the land deceptively, it was all legal."

"R.J.? Who is R.J.?"

"She's the lawyer. Oh, and she says her people lived in the kingdom."

"Who were her people?"

"I think she said the name is Casey."

Mother Rita looks over at me. "Well, I'll be. The Caseys. They did live in the kingdom. Luella was a Bobo. Once she married William, her name changed to Montgomery."

I scoop her hospital nightgown and robe into a pile. While she's resting, I'll do the laundry.

"All those families came here from South Carolina."

"So you've said."

"Half the land was registered in South Carolina in Robert Montgomery's name, and the other half was registered in Luella's name here in North Carolina. The original property straddled the two states."

"How do you know all this family history, Mother Rita? I couldn't find all those details in the library."

"Because my mama told me and her mama told her. Much as I love the historical record, it doesn't have all the answers, especially when it comes to our stories. Some history passed from mouth to mouth. Some history came down in the form of a mother's whisper."

But surely, I want to say, the more the story was retold, the more it changed. There is no way to verify all this. Once again I waver between skepticism and belief. So far Mother Rita has been right about a lot. And part of me knows there's truth to it. It's just her persistence to a rightful land claim that begs belief.

"Mother Rita, you remember that I'm leaving tomorrow, right?"

"They worked at the Oakland Inn for a widow woman. She needed them and they needed her."

"I've got to spend some time with Shawnie, not to mention I've got a house to sell. If I don't sell this house, I can't pay my bills."

"They saved up their money and bought the land. I always thought it was mighty modern of Luella's husband to put half the land in her name. I was told the kingdomfolk paid two hundred dollars. That was a lot of money back then." She looks at me brightly, as if I'm not even talking.

"Speaking of money, R.J. is going to represent you at your hearing. Do you have any savings to pay her? I'll try to contribute whatever I can." I think about Mama and wonder if she would be willing to help, if it comes to that.

"I reckon this land is worth millions today."

"So I hear." I study her. If Mother Rita is dying, I don't understand why getting the land back is so important to her. "Do you need money, Mother Rita? Is that what this is about for you?"

Her tone sharpens. "It's about dispossession. Look that word up, Miss Smarty-Pants."

I try to keep a straight face when all I want to do is scream. "Mother Rita, I'm just not sure how you can make a claim to the land. That cousin sold you out."

"Luella was smart. According to my mama, she was smarter than both of her husbands. Luella wouldn't have allowed all this land to be taken away like that. And don't talk to me about that cousin. The only person to blame here is Fred Thomas."

"Fred Thomas has been dead twenty years!"

"Good thing I don't have neighbors nearby. Wouldn't want them to hear you yelling at your grandmother."

I look down at the floor. "I'm sorry, Mother Rita. I didn't mean to raise my voice."

She gets up from the bed and begins to put the rest of her things away, talking as she moves.

"Luella had children, and she made sure they were educated. They had a school in the kingdom. Did you know that? They had schoolteachers and the kids went to school. The adults, too. The land provided for us, and my mother, Lily, was the first of our line to graduate from college. Bennett College for Women."

"Wait a minute. Your mother went to Bennett?" I am stunned. I'd never known we had any college graduates in the entire family line.

"Sure did. She was an education major."

"Nobody ever told me that."

She pauses and gives me another one of her strange smiles that

I've come to recognize as the joy she feels when talking about all this. "There are remnants, you know."

"Remnants of what?" I ask.

"The kingdom. There's a piece of the old schoolhouse still on the property. The palace where the king and queen lived is still back there."

"The palace? Wait a minute. Are there really remains of the kingdom on this property?"

"Yes, and you can't possibly leave before you see them. Maybe Maddie Mae's grandson can take you out there next week. I don't want you wandering off and getting lost again. There might even be hunters on the land this time of year. You'll probably hear their rifles going off. I put up no trespassing signs a while back and that seemed to work a little, but you still have to be careful."

I speak slowly: "So where is the palace?"

"Stephen can show you."

I don't have time to wait around for Stephen, and I don't relish the thought of walking through that brush, getting lost again. But Mother Rita is right. I need somebody who knows the terrain, who can navigate it without getting lost, not to mention I'm scared to death of snakes.

I know who can show me. The only person who can stop this eviction. I'll go see him, and then I will get on that plane to D.C. first thing tomorrow morning.

AL THOMAS'S HOUSE is easy to find. It's just down the road, and stickers spell T-H-O-M-A-S on his mailbox in metallic silver letters. When I pull into the driveway, he's outside washing his car. There are toys scattered in the yard.

"Al?" I call out.

He looks my way.

"I'm not sure if you remember me. I'm Nikki, Rita Lovejoy's granddaughter." I am going to have to hold back my anger when what I really want to do is tell him what he and his brother are doing to my grandmother is low-down and dirty.

He picks up the hose and rinses the soap from his car. "Course I remember you. How's your grandmother doing? I hear she's been over at Pardee for the last week."

The small-town grapevine is at it again. "She's doing better. Came home this morning."

A woman comes out holding a kitchen towel in her hands. "Hey, baby, who's our company?"

"Mrs. Lovejoy's granddaughter." He turns off the hose and slings a drying towel onto the car.

"Nikki Lovejoy-Berry," I say.

"Oh yeah. I heard you were here visiting. I'm Jessica, Al's wife. Want to come in for something cool to drink?"

I hesitate. I've got something serious to ask of Al and having a social visit with his wife isn't exactly part of the plan. But it would be rude to refuse her hospitality, especially with her smiling at me as if we're old friends. I glance at Al. He does need to finish washing his car before I can talk to him.

"That would be nice."

"I made iced tea this morning. It should be cold by now."

When we step into the house, two little boys sitting in front of a large-screen TV glance up at me.

"Lunch is ready," she calls out to them, but they don't turn around.

"Al never should've bought them that game. I could tell them the house was on fire and they'd say *okay* and keep playing."

"They sure are cute," I say. "I don't have any sons."

"Daughters?"

I sit at the kitchen bar and watch her wash up. She takes two glasses from the cabinet and fills them with ice.

"One daughter. She's nineteen."

"I guess we all want what we don't have. I wish I'd had a daughter. Instead, I live in a house full of people who leave the toilet seat up."

She is warm and so is her house. The floors are hardwood and covered in geometric contemporary rugs. A sectional sofa hugs the living room wall. The kitchen is open with stone countertops and high-end appliances. I quickly scan the room, eyeing the walls and fresh paint job. The house has been recently renovated, possibly within the last eighteen months.

"This tea is delicious."

"Thanks. I brew the tea myself and squeeze a little lemon in it."

"I just make mine from the packet. But yours proves the old-fashioned way is best."

She laughs. "Old-fashioned?"

"Sorry, I don't mean to be rude."

"Oh, I was just thinking of how I used to call this way old-fashioned when my mama made tea. Now I'm getting more and more like her."

"Don't we all?" I respond, though I sincerely hope I am not becoming my mother. It just seems like the right thing to say in the moment. I shift gears. "Jessica, I've got a question for you."

195

She taps the corner of her mouth with a napkin. "Alright, shoot."

"My grandmother says there used to be a kingdom on this land. You ever heard any of those tales?"

She leans over the counter, across from me. "Of course I have. Everybody around here has heard about that kingdom. The paper used to write articles about it all the time."

"You're from here?"

"Yes, I was born here. Then I went to school at Chapel Hill. That's where I met Al. I was the one who convinced him to move back home."

"You know, my grandmother's got nearly a half acre of flowers growing out there. Her garden is wondrous, really."

"I've bought flowers from her at the market before. No one can bloom a dahlia like Rita Lovejoy."

I look directly at her. I'm not sure if she knows anything about it, but as soon as I begin, I can tell she knows everything. "Jessica, I'll be honest. I'm here to talk to your husband about stopping the eviction."

She stands up straight, but her eyes are soft. "I'm so sorry, Nikki. This whole business puts a sour taste in my mouth. Your grandmother is a sweetheart."

Sweet isn't a word I'd use to describe Mother Rita.

"You should take him out on the land when you talk to him." She refills my glass. "He's better out there. Clearer."

I nod slowly.

"But you should also know that even if Al does agree, his brother jointly owns the land. He still lives in Durham and all he cares about is the money. He wants to split all the land up and sell off the lots."

She takes her glass and places it in the sink even though it's still half-full. I don't know how to respond to her kindness, so I just finish off my tea and thank her for the hospitality.

"Listen, how long are you staying? I want you to know you're always welcome. You like fondue? I host girls' night once a month and the next one is coming up. You're welcome to join us."

"I leave tomorrow."

"Oh, that's too bad. I make mine with a mix of Gouda and Gruyère cheese—"

Al appears in the doorway wearing his socks without shoes.

Jessica turns to him. "Honey, why don't you take Nikki out on the land and show her around?"

He regards me curiously, as if trying to read my thoughts. "She's already been out there. Not much else to see."

I'm suddenly grateful Mother Rita mentioned the remnants this morning. "My grandmother says there are parts of the kingdom still on the property. Some kind of palace? Do you know where I can find it?"

He glances at his wife and then back at me. "Give me a minute to change."

TWENTY-THREE

After Al changes into dry clothes and shoes and fetches his
hat, I waste no time hopping into his four-wheeler. He shouts
over the roar of the motor. "So you want to see the old kingdom?
There's not much left other than that old cabin!"

I'm afraid we'll get stuck and have to walk back, but he drives
the vehicle straight through what appears to be a sinkhole. I hold
on to the steel bar beside my seat.

We round a bend and come upon a two-story wooden house
that sits back from the path about a hundred yards. "Here we are.
This is where the king and queen lived. The locals say they called
it a palace, but I think that's just a rumor."

I get out of the vehicle. This is no mere rumor. This is the first
tangible evidence of the kingdom I've seen. And I believe with
every fiber of my being that it was their palace.

"It's safe to go inside. Last I checked, the wood was pretty
strong. One thing I can say, they knew how to build a house. Ain't
nothing in there, though, except for maybe some raccoons," he says.

For a moment, I've forgotten the main purpose of my visit is to talk to Al. I place one foot at a time on each step, testing for rotten boards. The front door swings open noisily. There are only two windows, so it's a little dark inside. I shine my cell phone flashlight. The stairs leading upstairs have disintegrated, but I trace out the first-floor layout with my steps. A bedroom on the back, a front living and eating area. To my right is a stone fireplace where some animal has built a nest and abandoned it. Cobwebs hang from the ceiling. The walls are set with mud, probably keeping the house warmer in winter. I estimate the entire first floor is six hundred square feet.

In the corner sits a dusty water pitcher. I close my eyes and imagine Luella here with her family, stirring something in a pot over the open hearth. In this house they ate and argued and made love, worried and celebrated, laughed and cried. I can feel them, not like ghosts or spirits, but like warmth. *Luella?* I call out in my mind and breathe deeply. The past has never felt more present for me. For a moment, I wish to be transported back in time, know what life was like for her in this house, but I remain in my body, planted on that floor even as a wave of light-headedness rushes over me. Standing in that house, I can feel the truth of Mother Rita's story with every hair on my body, what they gained, what they lost and sacrificed.

"What happened to all the other houses and cabins?" I ask as I come out, holding the pitcher in my hand. Seeing Al leaning so casually against his ATV makes my legs wobble as I descend the front porch. I'm caught between being angry at him for trying to evict my grandmother and unsettled by this house.

"At some point, they got torn down, I guess. I didn't even know this place existed before I moved back home."

"Is there anything else?"

We climb back into the vehicle and keep driving until we come to a clearing that appears to span a couple of acres. The grass is sparse; the land had obviously been cleared at one time. Al slows and turns off the motor.

"This is where they farmed. According to my wife they grew a lot of their own food. There's game around here, too. A lot of deer and wild turkey."

I try to imagine them working this field. It must have been so hard to scrape together a life anew. Together they could accumulate more and build more quickly. Working to feed their families. Distributing the fruits of their labor. Each person doing what they were able. No one yelling at them if they faltered, no man on a horse carrying a whip. I imagine them shaking off some of the sadness of their past as they reaped what was for them and them only, ate freshly grown vegetables rather than scraps, killed game and ate all the good parts roasted over a fire.

We drive past the field and push uphill. When we get to the top, there's only the remains of a chimney.

"They say this was the school for the children."

This is the schoolhouse Mother Rita talked about. "This is all that's left?"

"At least it's something."

This time, I've worn the right shoes, and I step surely through the scrubby brush as daddy longlegs scatter. I'm certain it gets cold up here in winter, and I imagine the children stoking the fire as the wood burned down to an ember. They would have fed it constantly so they could focus on their lessons. I wonder how many children lived in the kingdom, how they managed to learn with all of the ages together in one classroom, how many hours a day they studied before being called off to work for the rest of the afternoon.

I stand before the chimney in silence. A family tree isn't just something you draw on paper. It's an actual tree planted in the ground, with bark for skin and branches for arms. It's the earth pushed up into the sky. It's the physical manifestation of dreams, like the palace and the schoolhouse. A flame burns within me to know more. Queen Luella was a leader among leaders of this impossible settlement, and she'd been largely successful, so much that the land ownership had extended to nearly seventy years. This is why Mother Rita's desire to take back the land is so strong, so rooted in the stories her mother and grandmother passed down. Mother Rita's sense of aggrievement goes generations deep. Even Maddie Mae knows it. No wonder she was disgusted with how quickly I believed R.J. when she said there would be no recourse for getting the land back.

My grandmother isn't crazy. Far from it.

I turn on Al in a fury. "I know what you and your brother are doing."

He shakes his head as if to interrupt.

"You've got the power to stop this."

"There's nothing I can do," he says, looking at the ground.

"Yes, there is. You can stop the eviction."

"We've been sending her notices since April. She's had plenty of time to make plans. We've got a buyer and he wants the property free and clear."

"How can you do this? She's dying of cancer!" It hurts my heart to know Mother Rita received an eviction notice just after learning she was sick. I can see his body freeze up, and I know he has not heard this news. "Let her stay there until she dies. Please."

"We've been waiting to get this property ever since we learned we inherited the land eight years ago," he says. "My brother says he won't wait anymore."

"What?" A woodpecker starts rapping at something in the distance, and it's as if the constant *peck-peck-peck* is the tick of a clock. Eight years ago. "You inherited the land eight years ago? I thought your daddy died twenty years ago?"

"When Daddy died, we didn't even know he owned this land. He had just bought it months before his heart attack and nobody ever told us. We didn't learn we had inherited it until twelve years later. We were going to do something with the land but never got around to it. My brother says he's ready to sell now. He needs the money, and there's nothing I can do about it. I'm sorry, Nikki."

"Please, Al."

"Maybe your family can buy it?" he asks.

My eyes focus on him. "Buy back our own land? We've lived on this land for generations. It's *ours*." Somewhere in the back of mind I already know this conversation is a lost cause.

He looks down at his shirt, as if he is about to shrivel up.

I begin to walk away, clutching the pitcher to my chest.

"Come on, Nikki. Let me give you a ride back!" he calls out to me.

I don't know if I'll be able to find my way home without getting lost, but I do know that I'd rather eat dirt than get back on Al Thomas's vehicle.

ONCE I'M NEAR the house, I take my cell phone out of my pocket and dial R.J.'s office number, taking a wild chance that the lawyer will answer on a Saturday afternoon. To my surprise, she does.

"Hi, R.J., it's me, Nikki Lovejoy." I catch myself, surprised at how easily *Berry* disappears.

"Oh, Nikki, I meant to call you yesterday but got tied up in court. I found the land deed."

"Which one?"

"There's only one. My assistant scanned it in, and I'm going to forward it to you tonight. It's the deed of transfer between the Widow Davis and Robert and Luella Montgomery. Two hundred and five acres."

I'm not sure how the deed will help Mother Rita's upcoming court date.

R.J. continues on. "There's a bill of sale that says they paid two hundred dollars. One hundred thirty acres in North Carolina and seventy-five acres in South Carolina. The kingdom straddled the state line. Local legend has it they did that intentionally so they could flee to the opposite state if the law came after them. But I think that might be a myth. I believe there are two deeds. The one I found was registered in North Carolina. There should be another one down in Spartanburg, but somebody would have to actually travel down there to look."

"I'm sure Mother Rita would love to have a copy of that deed," I say.

"This won't help your grandmother get the land back, but I want to make an argument in court about her emotional connection to the land and why she has been so slow to move. I know the judge. She's a decent person and might respond well to that."

"I had a talk with Al Thomas. I thought I might convince him to delay the eviction while Mother Rita is sick."

"Good thinking. And what did he say?"

"He refused. Says his brother in Durham wants to sell and

there's nothing he can do to stop it." I don't mention how I'd just stormed off.

"Well, it was worth a try."

"I didn't know their daddy had been dead twelve years before they learned they had inherited the kingdom land," I say.

"If Fred Thomas didn't leave a detailed will or listing of his assets, that's possible."

"I see."

"Look, it's not uncommon for people to sit on land. Like I said before, it's wealth. You can borrow against it, lease it out, or just hold it and wait for the market to grow. I do wonder why they're finally ready to make a move now. Maybe the brother is in financial trouble. You never know. Our best hope is that we can get the judge to agree to let her stay there until death. Maybe your grandmother will be satisfied with that."

"Um, have you met Mother Rita?"

We both laugh, and my heart calms a little.

"I'm going back to D.C. tomorrow. But I wanted you to know that I appreciate all your help." I can see the back door now. Mother Rita's house really is charming, like a cottage out of a storybook. She is like an otherworldly fairy tending this land. I can't imagine her dying and leaving it behind. I'll return from D.C. for the hearing. I can't leave her in the middle of all this alone.

"You call me anytime, okay? And tell your grandmother hello from Doris Casey's granddaughter."

"I will."

I'VE BEEN GONE for a little over two hours, and from the sound of the television, I know Mother Rita is up and about.

I wash up in the bathroom and splash my cheeks with water. I haven't worn makeup since I arrived in Hendersonville, and my skin has tanned into an even brown. Mother Rita's style is rubbing off on me. Shawnie will be shocked. My flight leaves early in the morning. I need to text her so she can pick me up from the airport.

I call out to Mother Rita, and she responds that she's in the kitchen. She has documents in front of her, on her lap.

"Mother Rita, look what I found." I hold up the pitcher. "I just came back from—"

"Shh." She cuts me off with a whistle through her teeth. I hate it when she does that, but the sound is familiar to me now, so I obey. I can tell there's something she wants to show me. Maybe she has a copy of Luella's original deed that R.J. already found at the county office. Or maybe it's a death certificate, something that lists surviving children, giving me more names to add to our family tree.

Instead, I'm shocked when I see the red stamp across the top of the page Mother Rita passes to me. "I got another one," she says.

"But we haven't even been to court yet," I say as I read the paper.

Notice of Trespassing. 200 Lovejoy Lane. Rita Lovejoy. Please vacate the premises immediately. Any failure on your part to adhere to this order may be grounds for your arrest and prosecution for unlawful entry on property.

So the bulldozers have all but arrived.

TWENTY-FOUR

Luella

In the following years, things didn't change in a way you could see. But after the land was our own it was like we was reborn all over again. We was still working and scraping like we always done but now there was something happening on our insides. It wasn't like the fountain of joy and disbelief after freedom came, but it was close. Every morning sun promised new hope. Every fresh crop new belief. Every blessed child. Every creation by our own hands. We had set ourselves on a new path, and we could feel the grace of God in it.

After the deed was finally signed, we all gathered in the clearing, determined to walk as much of the land as we could. Just to lay eyes on it. *Oh, just to see his face!* That land was the face of God. Our God. And it spread over the mountain like a coat, ready to protect us from the storms. It kept the evil out. We had more land than we could wrap our arms around. We would grow and build and plant as far as we could and leave the rest to God's creatures.

In the early hours, we walked. Just looking and turning here and there. I held my Sunny's hand, quietly telling her what little I knew of the people who walked these hills long before us, who'd met at the river to trade. I told her how they followed the animals and kept close to the water. Picked wild plants. Carved rock into arrows. Answered to a chief rather than a king. I told her we had to remember them with every step. We might have held the deed, but this land was theirs. I couldn't help but be struck by the foolishness of property ownership while also knowing that without it, we was hopeless.

I suppose it wasn't no surprise that in the heat of our newfound joy, I grew with child again. As if to salute me, Robert touched my belly, which was barely swollen, his hand large enough to cover it. He dipped a cloth into a bowl of water and wiped my bare back, rested the moist toweling on my shoulder. I could feel his breath as I leaned back my head, cupping his cheek with one hand as he pressed his lips to the edge of my ear.

"Lu."

He hardened against me, and I let loose a moan. His hand went to my breast and stayed. A warmth flooded my thighs and I pressed them together. His skin was soft against mine. I had never been joined to Robert by God, but this tightness in my body, this unsteadying was a spirit thing. He was more than husband to me or father to our child, more than king. Robert was my awakening.

"Lu."

I pushed my back into his chest, hushing him. I couldn't bear this feeling. I had been bound to a master in childhood, then wedded to a man I didn't love, and now I was caught in a joining that threatened to steal my breath.

What good was life when I thought to lose him was to die?

Papa had not been able to love again after Mama died, and I understood that now. A need as strong as this was dangerous in a world like ours, where you could rejoice at night and weep in the morning. My body was mine now, but my feelings wasn't my own. What if they came again and took it all away? I wanted to push Robert aside, to protect myself from whatever hurt lay in store. But as he pulled up my skirt and moved to enter me, I was helpless to save myself.

IN 1880, WADE was born strong and loud. And though Sunny would always be his firstborn, the boy-child got in my Robert's spirit. Wade wasn't even three years old before Robert started daddy school. How to chop wood. How to square a corner. How to skin a squirrel. They walked that land round and round. And Sunny followed everywhere, unwilling to let her little brother learn nothing she didn't learn first. If Wade was a quick study, Sunny was quicker. When their daddy wasn't around, she taught her little brother letters, forcing him to carry her slate back and forth to the schoolhouse.

As the years went by, the children would stay at Papa's cabin whenever I went to town to sell liniment. Papa whittled toys, delighted them with his flute playing, made little slingshots they used to hurl rocks. Though we had a lot of newcomers who wasn't from Cross Anchor, us people in the original Zion's Travelers never let the kingdomfolk forget, including the children, that it had actually been Papa who had led us from his church to this mountain, not just the Montgomery brothers.

Papa enjoyed his grandchildren so much that he made the decision to turn over Sunday sermons to Reverend Couch. Papa was one of them preachers that knew the scripture by heart, having been made to listen to his master read to him every single morning since he was a boy. With a memory unlike any I've ever seen, he could quote scripture so accurate he'd dare you to look it up yourself. But Reverend Couch could read letters, and with the growing book smarts among the kingdom dwellers, Papa felt Couch could teach better.

Sometimes I thought Papa was fine, grateful just to be alive long enough to see the next generation of his flesh. In me, he had a daughter who would take care of him until the end of his days. In his grandchildren, he had immortality. Other times, I worried he was fading right before my eyes.

One April afternoon Papa stopped by the palace unexpectedly. The children was still at school and Robert was out working the crops. "Care to sit outside?" I asked. The spring air was warm enough for sitting.

"Better to be inside," he said.

I looked at him. Papa had something to say that wasn't for waggling ears. I let him in, and he sat in the armchair. The evening meal wasn't ready, but I had fresh bread to offer. Papa was thinner these days, and I wanted him to eat more. He took the loaf, and I poured water from the pitcher for both of us.

"What's on your mind?"

He finished chewing and swallowed. Ever since I could remember, my Papa had the manners of a gentleman.

"I got news about your husband."

I knew he meant William, not Robert, because he never called Robert my husband. I hadn't heard nothing lately, only that William was still sleeping in a house full of men. There was no new wife. No children. That's all I knew.

"It ain't bad news, is it?"

"Depend on how you see it."

So he wasn't dead. Papa never would have said that if he was. Nobody was waiting around for William to die. Robert still loved his brother, and I sure didn't hate him.

I finished the water in my cup, but it went down like a lump of flour.

"He coming back," he said.

"Back where."

"Here."

I sucked air through my nose, let it out softly. Surely Robert knew this already. He was the king. He knew everything first. He must've wanted Papa to tell me. For some reason, he couldn't. Why not? I wasn't going to scare.

"He coming back cause he sick, ain't he. More sick than he been."

He didn't answer.

"Why didn't Robert tell me? Why you here with this?" I couldn't stop the quick beating of my heart in my chest. It was like I was walking up a hill, but I was sitting right there in that chair, barely moving.

"Sometimes, I got to come to you as your papa. Other times I come to you as a man of God."

"And now?" I asked.

"I come to you as both, though you ain't asked my counsel."

"No, I ain't. But you giving it."

"He still your husband, Luella."

"I thought you said he wasn't no more. I heard you quote Corinthians."

"He sick and he need a wife to care for him."

"Seventh chapter, fifteenth verse, you said."

210

"What's right is right."

"What I tell my children, huh?"

"You got to talk to Robert. He having trouble with this, too."

"So I got to fix all the men."

"Luella, please."

The children ran in the door, smelling of the outdoors and the mule. "Wipe your feet!" I yelled too sharply.

I was mad at Papa for bringing me this news, because I already knew what it meant. I had to live with all my choices, the good and the bad. William was sick, and I wouldn't be the woman Papa raised if I didn't help him. Even if he wasn't my husband no more, I couldn't put a sick man out to pasture. There was a thing called duty.

I pulled the grass out of Sunny's hair. Wade climbed into his grandpa's lap and took a piece of bread from his fingers. Outside, the mule snorted over and over, as if trying to push something bothersome out her nose.

I DIDN'T KNOW how long it would be before William's return, but I knew me and Robert needed to talk about it. I waited a week after Papa's visit before I gathered myself enough to say something. The children was asleep and Robert was already in bed. I was preparing for the next day, so the candle was still lit. I could tell by the space of his breath he wasn't sleep. So I sat on the bed and rested a hand on his thigh.

"Robert," I said, not whispering or speaking loudly neither.

"Something wrong?"

"Why you ain't tell me your brother coming."

"What's to tell."

"What we going to tell the children? Where he going to live?"

"I'm sure he find a place. We got all this land. Maybe he live with your papa."

"Robert, how he going to live with Papa and he blind. Papa hardly handle his own self."

"William a grown man, Lu. He can find his way."

"A grown man who is your brother."

He sat up. "Don't you think I know that? How you think I feel? Here I am sitting on his throne, sleeping next to his wife, and being a daddy to his children?"

"They ain't his children. What's gotten into you?"

"Well, they should've been! Life ain't been kind to my brother!"

"Shh!" I put a finger to my lips, not wanting to wake Sunny and Wade. Now that I was looking at Robert, I knew this whole thing was hurting him bad as it was hurting me. The brothers had always been close, and the years and distance had not changed that. He was trying to figure out how to make space for William, same as I was.

I lay back and wrapped my body against Robert's backside. "We figure it out. We make sure William alright." I had no idea how we would do this, but I couldn't let Robert know how uncertain I was, how uneasy William's return made me.

TWENTY-FIVE

W e didn't have much time to consider things because William arrived at our front doorstep two weeks later.

Robert was out working with the men in the fields when William knocked on the door. The children was gone to the schoolhouse, and I was fixing my bag to go meet Jola and Rachel. When I opened the door, William was standing on the porch, facing the lane. I almost didn't recognize him from behind. His hair was completely white, his shoulders narrow. But it was the same long neck and straight back. And there was a traveling bag next to him.

"William?"

He turned an ear toward me. "Luella?"

I placed both my arms around his waist. I could feel his thinness, like paper. When he turned to press his cheek to mine, I caught the scent of rotting teeth.

"Come on, let me help you."

I guided him by the hand inside and led him to the chair, noticing that he walked with a stick. It had been almost a decade since I'd seen him last, and he looked old—not older but old. I was surprised and it showed. Wasn't no need to hide it since he couldn't see my face. "I like what you done with the place," he said, turning his head.

"You ain't been here five minutes and you already fooling with me."

"That chair over there is new."

I sat down across from him. "I thought they said you was blind."

"I can still see a little. The world ain't all dark."

I considered that for a moment.

"At night, it's different. But I see that chair over there. And I see you." He looked straight at me.

"I don't know what to say."

Both of us was quiet for a moment, but we wasn't lost for words. It was as if there was too many words, so our tongues rested.

Finally, he said, "You happy, Luella?"

I couldn't answer that without feeling bad, but William's ear was turned to me and I knew he could hear if I lied. So I answered truthfully.

"Yes, I am."

"What's the children's names?"

"Cordelia and Wade. We call the girl Sunny."

"Sunny. I like that." I didn't sense anger from William. Not sadness neither. Maybe he was here to discover what could've been.

"Why did you leave us, William?"

He slipped a twig out of his pocket and used it to scratch the back of his head. When he was done, he slipped it back into his pocket. Finally, "I was trying to build your schoolhouse."

"You was trying to what?"

"I wanted to surprise you. I wanted to do it on my own. But then I got hurt."

I managed to say "No one told me" even while my throat was closing up.

"I sent the money."

William should have told me he'd gone to the mines to earn money to help with the schoolhouse. He should've just asked the council instead of doing it on his own. He was the king. I wanted to say all this, but my throat wouldn't open. Robert hadn't told me that, and his betrayal was choking me, too.

"Don't blame my brother," William said, sensing my anguish. "I gave him my blessing. And wasn't that a good thing? Y'all got children now. God's greatest gift."

Weeks of waiting for word from William. Robert delivering the news his brother wasn't coming back. The proposal. The night I took Robert to be mine. The trust I put in both these men. The so-called honor of being queen. I wanted to burn that crown.

"You was my husband, William!"

"I was so shame, Luella. I didn't treat you like a man ought to treat his wife. And I couldn't let you take care of me after that."

I shook my head.

He stretched his left leg out in front of him, slowly, carefully, as if this conversation hurt his body. I didn't want this apology.

But he had gone to work in the mine to earn money for the school-house.

I got up and walked to the cupboard. "When you take your pants off tonight, rub this on your leg."

He held the jar in the palm of his hand, carefully, as if he was holding a treasure. "I will do that, Luella." The way he said my name reminded me of our early days of courtship. "I heard about this liniment."

"Where you staying?"

"George brought me, but his place ain't big enough, so I don't know yet."

"You stay here till you figure it out," I said, speaking and thinking at the same time. I didn't know how Robert would handle him staying at our house, and I still hadn't told the children about their uncle. But I couldn't just make William leave. He didn't have nowhere to go. And while there was most likely space in somebody's cabin, conversations needed to happen between me and him first.

"We got plenty room here," I found myself saying.

The children came home before Robert, and I met them outside on the porch. I told them their daddy's brother would be staying with us a spell, but I didn't say he was also my husband. They was young enough that no one had told them their daddy had a brother so that was enough news to excite them. I made them sit before their uncle William, and I listened along with the children as William wove stories of the mine and the accident that nearly blinded him completely. As he talked, I watched him. He could make out some things, just enough to get around with his stick. And his listening was alert—when the children moved around the room, he moved his head with them. More than once, I saw him turning his head to listen. William had always been smart, and he used that intelligence in this new body.

I took a careful survey of him. It wasn't just his leg that ailed him. His whole left side looked weak, from his cheek to his arm down to his foot. He would need help. And as his wife before God, I had no choice but to provide it.

TWO THINGS CHANGED that week. William moved in with us and my monthly didn't come. That meant there was five of us living in that house with one likely on the way. But there was another number. I went from one husband to two. William moved his things to the upstairs room, sharing with Wade, but sat with us for dinner each night. In the meantime, I didn't tell Robert about my missing blood.

The children was noisy all the time, still excited about our new houseguest, an uncle they'd never met. Two weeks after William's arrival, I readied the table, watching the brothers together for the first time in years. This had not been a planned reunion, and though the air was uneasy, I could sense them wading through the muck.

"Brother."

"Brother."

They had never called each other by name; at least that hadn't changed. Robert settled in his seat. "I hear the men up the way got room. Maybe you can stay with them."

William answered slowly. "It's a lot of places on the mountain. Shouldn't be no trouble for me to find a bed."

The brothers eyed one another, but the children's questions broke the chill.

"You got more brothers, Daddy?" Wade asked.

"I had a lot of them. They're all gone now."

"Gone where?" Sunny asked.

"Y'all eat up."

"What about you, Mama?"

"No brothers or sisters."

"And your mama died when she gave birth to you?"

"Hush now. Eat up like your daddy say." The children glanced curiously between me and Robert, as if they was just now realizing we'd been children once. Questions about the past when you'd come from where we come from never ended in simple answers and sometimes didn't end with answers at all.

Meantime, the men ate.

"William tried the liniment," I said.

When Robert looked at me with a question in his eye, I remembered I had always rubbed the liniment on him. Back, legs, feet. Of course, I hadn't done that with William, though I saw how Robert might assume. I tried to answer his unspoken question. "You rub it on your legs, William?"

"It was good. Thank you, Miss Luella."

I picked up the mashed potatoes. "More?" I asked William. It was customary to offer the guest first, but Robert was the man of the house. And whether or not William counted as a guest was questionable, especially since he'd built much of this house with his own two hands. No matter which way I stepped, a big old hole waited for me to stumble.

"Brother, you first," William said, gesturing to Robert. The younger brother didn't respond, so I put a little bit on his plate anyway.

A few minutes more of us eating in silence. How to mark the time? Forks clanking, the mule whinnying, trees rustling, a fly that refused to settle.

After dinner, William retired to his room and Robert sat in his chair. He didn't say nothing, and I knew, with the certainty of a wife, to leave both men be.

AS THE DAYS went on, I found myself enjoying William's company. He was kinder, gentler than he'd been before. When me and the children acted awkward with him, he corrected us gently, reminding us he could hear better than most and his sight wasn't completely gone. He refused to allow us to treat him as helpless. He had learned to be useful in that house of men, and he did the same in my house. He swept out the front room and porch each morning, wiped down the table after we ate, made the bed and tidied the room he shared with Wade. William cleaned enough that I didn't have to anymore.

We was mindful not to move things around. He struggled with his left leg, but now he moved through the house almost as quick as I did. He liked to walk through the kingdom, greeting old friends, learning the names of strangers, using his stick to guide him. The council invited him to join again, and he walked with Robert to council meetings on the full moon, the younger brother guiding him by the elbow. The sight heartened me that they might come together again as brothers one day.

William surely sensed his brother's distress, but he didn't respond and I didn't push it. I felt a duty to my first husband, to honor the vows I'd made to God. That's what Papa had told me. I had to work this out, and I was doing my best.

One morning, two months after William arrived, I overheard the two of them on the porch talking. It was the most I'd heard them say to each other since William came back. Wade was outside with them, so I knew their words was taking the youngster's ears into account.

"I found a place for you to stay," Robert was saying.

"I got a life right here. Wade, you don't mind me staying in your room, do you?"

"No, sir."

"This is my life, brother. It ain't yours no more."

"You don't got to worry. The feelings between me and Luella done dried up. She like a sister to me now."

"Brothers and sisters don't live together. They each go their own way."

"There's plenty room. What's eating you?"

"You eating me."

I stepped outside. "Wade, baby, come in the house." After I made sure he was all the way upstairs in his room, I crept back downstairs to listen.

"We family. And this how you treat me?" I heard William's voice crack. I needed to do better at reminding Robert there wasn't no more love between me and William. This was my fault. But I'd been sick with this baby.

I stepped outside. William sat slack in the rocker, but Robert was leaning forward, as if ready to spring. "Robert."

"Lu, are you my wife or his?"

"Robert, stop talking crazy. We agreed we would help him."

"When did we agree that, Lu?"

"I'll go pack my things." William pushed up out of his chair.

"No, you won't," I said. William needed to leave, but not like this. I didn't want to be the cause of these brothers hating each other.

"Lu," Robert said. "I can't live like this."

"It ain't forever, Robert. Give it time. He our family."

"Our family?"

"He our . . . he my . . ." I stopped. I didn't know what word to use. William had called me a sister, but really we was more than that to each other. I felt a tenderness toward William, perhaps stronger now than when we'd been together. It was as if I could see him better now. He looked toward me, as if he could see me, too.

TWENTY-SIX

O ne afternoon, I met Robert by the creek where he usually took his midday rest. I sat beside him and spread my dress out around me. There had been so much tension in the house that I still hadn't told him he would be a daddy again. Today I planned to surprise him with the news and gift him a bag of chestnuts. "You feeling alright today?"

"Yeah," he answered without asking me the same.

During the coldest days of winter, the creek froze, but now it trickled downstream and I could hear some women laughing as they filled their buckets. This clear stream was our source of drinking water, and we respected it. We'd managed to avoid sickness because of some of our practices. We'd been told that the ones who lived in the area before us had met on this mountain for trading, sleeping near the creek for a few nights before returning to their homes. We tried to treat the creek with the same respect they had.

Robert must have been thinking about these old stories, too, because he said, "My daddy said in Africa our people climb trees high as the sky."

"Ain't no such thing as a tree that reach the sky, Robert."

"Back home, there is. And the men from our tribe was tall enough to see over them."

"Imagine a man being tall as all that."

"Not just the men."

"I sure hope Sunny don't get too tall to find a husband."

"He said where we come from, some of the women lean down to kiss the men."

"He said that?"

"That's what my daddy told me."

"But your mama wasn't from there. So maybe Sunny got a chance."

He turned his head toward me, as if I wasn't understanding a thing he was saying.

"I know it ain't been easy, this thing with your brother. He just need a soft place to rest his head for a minute. He'll leave our place in due time," I said.

"Due time."

"Robert."

"I see the way he look at you."

"Stop talking foolish. He blind."

"A man see with more than his eyes."

"William and me is still making our peace. I owe him that."

"And what you owe me?"

I placed a hand in his. He didn't pull away, but his skin was cold and limp against mine. He'd dropped a half-eaten apple on the ground, and a fly nibbled at it. "Robert, why didn't you tell me he went to the mines for me? To earn money and build the school-house I asked about."

I had thought so many times on how to ask him this question.

Waiting allowed my anger to settle so I could ask it calmly. Being pregnant gave me patience.

He stood. "See, that's it, Luella. I ain't your husband and I never was!"

It was impossible to remain on the ground with a man like Robert standing over you, so I pushed up, too. "Answer the question, Robert."

He lowered his voice to a whine. "You making me choose between you and the only brother I got left. Don't you know how hard this is for us?"

"You talking nonsense. You should have told me William was working to send money for the schoolhouse."

"I need you to choose."

"Robert, I came down here to tell you some news."

"The only thing I want to hear from your lips is that you hear what I'm saying."

I couldn't stand to hear him begging like this. I bent my chin to my chest and wiped my eye. Of course I chose Robert. I would tell William to leave. But the words wouldn't form on my lips, and the bag of chestnuts lay forgotten on the ground.

THAT EVENING, WHEN we was all seated around the table eating our dinner, William said, "I been meaning to congratulate you, brother."

"For what?"

William clapped his hands together. "I know you ain't going to believe this, but I'm happy you give Luella children. She a good mother."

I stopped chewing and stared at William in disbelief.

"I hope you get another girl smart as that Sunny. Do you know she can count all the way to a hundred?"

Robert's neck swiveled, and his eyes fixed on my belly. Sunny broke out in a counting singsong, and Wade pushed her on the arm.

"I want a brother!" Wade declared. "So me and him can be like you two."

"I was going to tell you earlier today at the creek," I said softly.

"How long you knowed?" Robert asked quietly.

"Not long. I don't know how William picked up on it. How you pick up on it, William?" My voice shook.

"You run to that outhouse every few minutes. That's a sign, ain't it? I been around pregnant womenfolk before." He paused, understanding clouding his face. "Brother, you didn't know?"

This didn't feel right. We should have been praying gratitude over this baby. Instead, my husband was looking at me with distrust on his face. And here William was as jubilant as if the baby was his. It was Robert looking like he suspected he might not even be the daddy. I was living with two husbands and this was the cost. In the mornings and evenings, two men ate at my table. At night, I heard the snores of the one beside me and the coughs of the other one upstairs. Robert hadn't touched me since William arrived, but this baby had been made before this turn in our lives.

Something had to change, but I felt powerless to do it.

THE SPIRIT GOT a way of moving heavens and earth when we too weak to do it our own selves. Papa used to say that when I was little. He used to rely on that belief when it came to the way white men treated us. We was too weak to fight back against guns and dogs, so the Spirit took care of it. But sometimes the Spirit brought dark times and heartache, too.

Robert didn't speak to me for two days after he learned from his brother that his wife was having another baby. On the third night of silence, I woke up with wetness between my legs.

"Robert, Robert." I shook him.

He sat up and turned to me. "What is it?"

"Something ain't right."

He pulled back the cover. Through the window, the moonlight shone bright enough to reveal a dark stain spreading across the bed. He sprang up.

"I go get Jola. Lay back. Stay right here!"

He struggled to pull on his boots. "Stay still, Lu. I get you help. Sunny, wake up! Come see about your mama and I'll be right back. Sunny, come on now!"

I did as I was told and waited for my daughter to come downstairs. But when a searing pain hit me in my back, I screamed.

TWENTY-SEVEN

I asked God to tell me something. What did this squabble between husbands mean when my baby died in my belly before it had feet to stand on?

It had been months since I lost the baby, and William was still living in our house. Robert would leave before sunup, when the rooms was still dark and he didn't have to talk to his brother. I would awaken next so I could rouse the children for school. Sunny and Wade didn't like waking up early in winter, but now that it was spring, they was easier to manage. We still shared a dinner that came out of the kingdom kitchen in the evening, but Robert had finally installed a cookstove in our house, and in the coldest months I used it in the morning for breakfast. Robert stacked fresh wood outside the door.

That morning, I kept it simple with hot water bread and heated water for coffee. William had never drunk coffee before he moved down to the mines, but now he had a taste for it. I liked it sweetened with just a bit of sugar. He liked it bitter.

I walked the children to the schoolhouse, and by the time I returned he was sitting at the table sipping from his cup. I sat across from him. I had things to do. I'd promised Jola I would go on the delivery with the women that morning. They'd be loading the wagon and departing before long. But I stayed in my spot, every part of me wanting to go back to sleep.

"Taste good," he said.

"Glad you like it."

"I been asking around about a spare bed."

"You built this house, William."

"And I walked out of it."

"I don't harbor no feelings about that no more," I said truthfully. I didn't have room for more feelings. All of mine was tied up inside my chest.

His voice softened. "Yes, you do. And I understand it. Wasn't right of me to leave here without saying goodbye."

"You did say it. I just wasn't listening."

"Did I? I planned to come back."

"You sure about that? Let's say you hadn't got hurt. Let's say you worked. You sent the money for the schoolhouse. You would've come back after that?" As soon as I uttered the question, I regretted it. It was a child's question. Not something that ought to pass from a grown woman's lips.

He didn't say nothing. I thought of what life would've been like without my children, living in this big house with just William. I loved Sunny and Wade. They was my heart. But motherhood was the kind of thing that you had to experience to know if it suited you or not. Now I knew. Losing my baby had been like losing an arm I ain't know I had. Just the mere memory of all that blood quickened my heartbeat.

227

William tried to get up but lost his balance somehow. I rushed to his side and held his arm. He leaned into me, and though he was thinner than he'd been before, he felt wiry and strong. He was still the man who'd led us up that hill and shared his last drop of water with me.

He put an arm around me, but instead of using me for support, he pulled me to him.

"I know this a little late coming, but I want to say I never should've laid a hand on you. I had a lot of time to think down there at the mines. When I come back and you didn't hate me, it was like water rushed over my neck. Joy like I ain't felt in a long time."

"Course I don't hate you. But I appreciate the apology." I rested my head on his chest.

We walked over to the chair, and I held his elbow while he sat down. I sat across from him, fully aware that I was likely to miss the trip to town with the women that day.

"I'm sorry about your baby."

This was his first mention of it, but the hurt was still fresh. All I could do was nod.

"But you got two fine ones. That girl Sunny is one and a half. She remind me of you."

"That's what Papa say."

We sat in silence again. I tucked my hands together, gazing off at nothing. Sitting with William was comfortable. There was no awkwardness in it, just like in the early days. He closed his eyes.

"What's it like?"

"Being blind?" he asked.

"No. Being alone." I had never been alone. Even though I hadn't had a mama, I'd had Papa. Then I'd had William. Now

Robert. And the children. With the baby gone from my belly, I could feel surges of loneliness, mostly at night when everybody was sleep. But I was never alone as he had been down at the camp.

He sighed. "It ain't easy. But I got my memories. I remember my parents. My granddaddy. They was good people. I had brothers and sisters. My folks told us stories of our home."

"Africa just a dream," I said. "Don't nobody remember. And if they do, it's all jumbled."

His eyes opened, and he seemed to be staring straight at me. "No, it ain't no dream. Their memories was clear as day."

"But do we really know it was kingdoms? Maybe that's made up."

He shook his head. "Africa had kingdoms, Luella. That's a fact. I know we left behind something real. They took away our culture, our traditions, but they didn't take all our memories."

"So you wanted to come up this mountain and try to capture Africa?"

"Why not?" His nostrils flared. "What else was there? Down in Cross Anchor, we wasn't really free. We was just living a nightmare with no end."

"You sound like Robert."

He grunted, and I wasn't sure if he was pleased with that comparison or not. I thought of all the ways we'd struggled up in these hills, how hard it had been to scrape together a life. We'd had to pay our way out from under the law. We'd had to buy the land or remain in debt to the Widow and possibly be kicked off after her death. At every turn we'd had to do something miraculous to survive.

"The young people don't understand. Some of them leave and don't come back."

"Y'all got to tell the story," he said. "So they remember."

"What story? The story of how the Klan run us off? The story of how they accuse us of eating our own, how they beat the men if y'all dare vote?"

He nodded. "They can't grab on to the strength if we don't share the pain."

"You a good leader, William."

"Sometime I think I'm a fool."

"You ain't never been a fool."

"Except when I left you."

He moved his leg, and I saw that it agonized him. I slid out of my chair and knelt at his feet. I pulled off his slipper and his sock. His foot was swollen on the side of his big toe.

"How long your foot been like this?"

"A week."

I rubbed it. "Do this hurt?"

He let out a grunt in answer. I took off his other shoe and put both feet in my lap, rubbing the sore spot. He moaned.

"You need a—"

The door opened behind us. Robert stood in the doorway, his mouth open as if mid-sentence. Then his lips closed and he just stared. I knew what he saw. His wife kneeling on the floor rubbing his brother's feet, my dress pooled around me, his brother's eyes closed, head leaned back.

"Robert, what you doing home?"

"I could ask the same of you."

"What?" That was all I could say. Robert knew I had planned to go into town with the women. He must've seen them leave and believed I was with them.

"I been looking everywhere for you. It's your papa."

"My papa?" I dropped the feet out of my lap and stood.

I didn't look back at William before rushing past Robert, but I had a bad feeling. Somehow I knew I was leaving one storm to go see about another.

SOMETIMES WHEN A tree fall don't nobody know why. There ain't been no rains to loosen the roots. No storms to unsettle. No sign of rot on the bark. No brittle branches. No holes in the leaves. No telltale lean.

When Papa fell, it was like that tree. One minute he was laughing and making toys for my children, and the next he was on the forest floor. And all of us left with a gap where the chilly wind could blow right through.

I thought back to the conversation we had before coming up that hill, when Papa sat me down and talked to me like a woman. Not like a flower to be pollinated by a husband, but like a decision-maker. He'd come to me with a *what if*. At the time I'd understood he was asking for my blessing. He hadn't wanted to make that move if I wasn't fine with it.

I thought of that last conversation me and Papa had before William came back from the mines, when Papa came to me once again and talked to me like a woman. I had been less than respectful, had even thrown his own scripture in his face. I regretted that moment, and with Papa's body freshly prepared for burial but still between the sky and the earth, I recounted every moment I'd ever had with him that made me less than proud. If I had him one more day, I'd hold him tight. I'd listen even when my ears ached.

The women brought me food. They kept my children when all I could do was sit and remember.

I wondered, when I thought of all the men in my life, how a body could measure up to the kind of respect Papa granted me. Would Sunny have it. Would Wade give it to the woman he loved. Would the husbands who still lived in the kingdom, and the ones who had moved on with their families elsewhere, go to their women and ask for their blessing in all things that mattered to the family.

On the day we laid Papa to rest, in a grove where we had marked all of our lost ones with rocks, I stood between Robert and William. When I was young, I'd barely been able to determine which brother I liked better. So I'd gone with the one that passed me his canteen, who built me a house they called a palace, who gave me a crown and called me queen.

But now I gazed up at Robert, knowing that he was the one, the only one who had honored me the way my papa had. I couldn't remember a decision we hadn't made together. How had I missed his devotion? Out of duty to a husband who had abandoned me, I had lost sight of the love that meant more to me than life.

Reverend Couch spoke the kindest words about his friend and fellow man of God. The men of the council led a low hymn in deep tones, the women joining and creating a harmony that stilled us all. One by one, the children placed flowers on top of Papa's box. I wished for a hand in mine, though neither brother offered.

When the service ended, I knew what to do. After the libations had been poured, after the scripture was read, after the tears was dried, after the children was put to bed and William was snoring, I would claim Robert as my true husband, do what I wish I had done when William first came back and my papa was still alive. Papa had only wanted me to make it right, not cause more confusion.

In our bed, under the same covers where we'd said our private vows, I pressed into Robert's back and spoke, knowing he was awake and could hear me. I whispered I was sorry, that I would ask his brother to leave, that I would honor him the way he had honored me.

What I didn't count on was the hurt on top of hurt, the grief on top of grief I would feel when he turned to me and said, softly, quietly, in my ear before pressing his lips into my wet cheek, that it was too late for us.

PART

THREE

TWENTY-EIGHT

Nikki

I make the difficult decision to return to D.C. Sunday morning, telling myself that it's because I don't want to pay the change fee for the flight. The truth is, I'm running away. When Shawnie arrives at the airport to pick me up, I hug her to me tightly. We didn't talk much while I was gone, and I've missed her so much it hurts my stomach. She doesn't hug me back.

"You look different," I say, and I mean it. It has only been a week, but she has cut her shoulder-length hair into a curly bob. She's wearing a pair of my earrings, and her outfit looks vaguely familiar, too. It strikes me that overnight she has blossomed from a shy high school graduate into a young woman.

She fingers my earrings. "I didn't think you'd mind if I borrowed them."

I wonder if I, too, look different. After all, I'm the one who has encountered the history of a hundred years in the past week. Inside, I'm probably someone entirely new. In addition to the news that we are descendants of an actual queen, I have a grandmother now, a real flesh-and-blood grandmother, not just someone who sends a card on holidays and visits D.C. every blue moon.

With all the traffic, it's going to take us a while to get home, and I'm not prepared to tell everything, not just yet. But Shawnie has no idea about the knots in my stomach, so she asks, "How's Mother Rita?"

I want to tell Shawnie about the cancer, but I need to talk to Mama first. I don't want to lie to my daughter. I'm so weary of secrets. At first, my lips refuse to move.

"She's not great," I manage to say.

"Why? What's wrong?" Shawnie isn't looking at me, but I can tell from the tension in her hand that grips the steering wheel, she's listening closely.

"I'll fill you in later. First, I want to get something to eat. My stomach is grumbling." I smile to lift the mood.

I have so much to tell her about Mother Rita. How she checks out ten books from the library at a time. How the morning light falls over the mountain in a gray mist and the dahlias appear to wait for her to walk out there before peeking at her through their buds. How she returns to the house ravenous for a hot breakfast after working outside all morning.

"I didn't tell Grandma you went down there. She thinks you were at a conference," Shawnie says.

I compelled Shawnie to keep this secret from Mama, recklessly cornering her into withholding information from the woman we both love, and she has not only kept it from Mama, she has made up a lie. And now, knowing what I know, that my grandmother never stopped loving any of us, I'm ashamed. It's time for all of us to lay down our armor, even if we've worn it so long it has become second nature.

EVER SINCE MAMA walked in the door, she has been talking. *I found a Christmas cruise and I'm thinking about going with some friends, what do you think? The weather this summer has been brutal. Did you see the mayor appointed a new schools chancellor? If I get one more ticket from those speed cameras, I'm giving up my car and taking the Metro from here on out.* Mama always chats like this when we haven't seen each other for a few days. It's like she saves up her words for me. She has taken off her shoes, and her feet are wrapped beneath her. She rubs one foot absentmindedly. We're sitting across from one another on the sofa in my apartment. Finally, looking around, she says, *You need to get a housekeeper in here. I'm getting too old to clean for you.*

Mama's need for order is stifling sometimes. I am not the messiest person nor am I the neatest. She'd approved when Darius and I moved into this low-rise apartment building just a couple of years after we married, planning to put down our roots in this D.C. neighborhood filled with older residents who kept their yards pristinely trimmed and delivered food after my daddy died and shouted from the porch when someone's guest unknowingly parked in their favorite street parking space. After Darius moved out, Mama asked for a key and it was a relief to give it to her. For years, it was nice to come home to clean rooms and a hot dinner waiting for me and Shawnie.

"Mama," I whisper when she finally stops talking long enough for me to begin. I'd hoped I could speak to her while Shawnie was out, but she is still in her room. "You doing okay?" I'm stalling because I'm nervous.

"I'm doing fine. My left foot has been hurting me, but the

doctor says the diabetes is under control." Mama goes to yoga three times a week. She may have type 2 diabetes, but she's fitter than I am.

"You been keeping up with your blood sugar?" I ask.

"I do everything I need to do."

"Except change your diet."

"You don't know what I do."

I sigh. This is an old conversation that has been replayed too many times to count. Mama is stubborn, and that's a fact. She's convinced she knows more than the doctors. But with the news of Mother Rita's illness, I want all of us to take better care of ourselves.

I lower my voice, as if by speaking quietly I can soften the blow. "Mama, I wasn't at a conference last week. I've been in Hendersonville."

I expect her to ask me what I was doing down there. She doesn't.

Instead: "How's she doing." She says this without hesitation, as if she hasn't spent the past eight years nursing a wound. She doesn't lift her voice, doesn't indicate her level of curiosity by looking me in the eye. It's almost as if she doesn't care whether I respond or not. But I know she cares, because she wouldn't ask it otherwise.

"She's sick."

"How sick?"

I decide to deliver it straight. There really is no other way. "It's cancer."

She's quiet. I can tell she's taking in the news. "How bad is it?"

This time, it's a real question. "Bad, Mama. She spent a few days in the hospital while I was there, but she's home now."

"How did she seem?" She isn't looking directly at me, but I'm sure she's watching me out of the corner of her eye.

"You wouldn't even know. She's refused chemo."

Finally, "What made you go down there, Nikki?"

I still can't explain it. The sudden phone call. The quick decision to accept the invitation. "She called and asked me to come."

She grimaces, as if processing that Mother Rita called me instead of her.

"I grew up in that house. Played in that yard and helped in the garden. We sold flowers every weekend," she says, staring at nothing.

"You never told me anything about selling flowers."

"My daddy and his brothers built that house with their own hands."

"My great-grandmother graduated from Bennett College."

"When I left Hendersonville, I vowed never to move back. I hated it there."

"Not only did you deny me, but you denied Shawnie."

"All throughout high school I couldn't wait to leave."

"How could you, Mama?"

"I felt like I was suffocating down there."

"You never said a single word about a kingdom or a queen or any of that."

She swivels her head to look at me.

"And Mother Rita's been dealing with this sickness all by herself," I say, the words tumbling out. "That on top of the eviction notice."

She drops her feet off the couch so suddenly that I think for a moment she's about to run out the door. But she stills, barely moving.

"What eviction notice?"

"The Thomas family is kicking her off the land. There's a court date—"

"A court date?" She gets that look she gets whenever she is furious. But her eyes are trained on me, as if I've done something wrong.

"Yes, Mama. They've issued a notice to vacate the premises. I tried to talk to Al Thomas, but he says—well, anyway, we hired a lawyer to handle it."

She leans in, as if to examine me. "What on earth are you talking about, Nikki? You spoke with Albert Thomas? You hired a lawyer?"

"Yes."

"They never expressed any interest in the land in all these years. It must be worth something now."

"Mama, it's worth millions. Wait, how do you know about that?" Now it's my turn to look incredulous. She hasn't spoken to Mother Rita in a long time.

There's so much I need to say to her, but I don't even know where to begin. I can't understand how the two of them could waste all these years not speaking or seeing each other. I can hear Shawnie moving around in her room and worry she'll come out any second and interrupt us.

I suck in a breath. "You never let me and Shawnie get to know her and then you cut her off. And now there's no time left!"

"I'm so sorry, Nikki." I can see now that she's crying. But I hurt, too.

"How could you do this?"

I wait, but she says nothing. It's the same old, same old. Mama shutting down when I try to get something out of her. Mama putting everything into the boxes inside her head and closing the lid. My voice returns to a whisper. "Ever since Daddy died, we haven't been the same. He wouldn't want this for us, Mama. He wouldn't want us to break apart."

She wipes at her eyes with the back of her hand. I don't move to get her a tissue. I'm tired of taking care of everybody's feelings.

"We need therapy. You know that, right?" I've never been to therapy in my life, but if there is a family that's a candidate, it's ours.

"I can't argue with that," she says with a hollow laugh.

Shawnie comes out of her room wearing earbuds and a backpack. She doesn't bother to speak to either of us before walking out the front door, turning the key in the lock behind her.

TWENTY-NINE

The next morning is Monday, and I arrive at the office early. I've got to make some headway on this house and return my clients' phone calls. Darius has shown the house twice since I've been gone, but I need to put together a walk-through tour for my social media and send a few texts to other agents. I'm texting with my photographer when Darius sets a Starbucks cup on my desk.

I look up at my ex-husband, the kind of guy who makes casual jeans look like office wear. He was the one who got me into real estate, and honestly, he's better at it than I am. He's charming, smart, and aggressive—all traits that work for him.

He sits on the edge of the desk inside my tiny shared office. "Welcome back. Those clients of yours were about to drive me crazy."

"I owe you one."

He nods toward my phone. "You're wasting your time marketing the house at that price."

"I'm letting everyone know that I'm entertaining all offers," I say.

"The clients will never agree to it, but it's the right move."

I look up at him, sigh, and put the phone down. It has been nearly six years since the divorce, and Darius and I have managed to make our way through the shift, co-parenting Shawnie with relative ease. Neither of us has remarried, so that makes it simpler. He had a few girlfriends in the early years, but the most recent one seems to be the real deal. They've been dating for close to three years, and neither seems to mind the constant questions about when they're planning to make it official. Though my feelings for Darius have changed over the years and I would never be jealous, I do sometimes envy their easy companionship.

I scratch my scalp. Vaguely, I remind myself I need to get my braids redone.

"You okay?" he asks.

"Yeah, why do you ask?"

"You look a little sad."

That was the same thing Bryan said. Why does everyone think I look sad? I haven't been able to slow down long enough to take inventory of my feelings. I'm just putting out fires as best I can.

"Hey, I have a question to ask you," I say.

He grabs a chair from an empty desk and seats himself next to me.

I tell him everything that's going on with Mother Rita, and he listens attentively, only interrupting to ask a few questions. Though he's familiar with title searches and the importance of establishing chain of title, just as I am, he only knows generally about Black people losing land through predatory measures.

"First, I'm sorry to hear about your grandmother. That has to be tough after all you've been through."

"Just help me figure this out, please."

"Alright, chill, Nikki. I'm only trying to show some sympathy."

"Sorry." I try to calm myself. "I'm just stressed. But what do you think we can do to get the land back?"

He pauses. "Now that I think about it, I read in the newspaper something about heirs' property. I think the name was Reels. Two brothers in North Carolina who were jailed for refusing to leave their land."

"Jailed? Darius, are you serious?"

"Of course, that won't happen to your grandmother. Didn't you say she has a good lawyer? I can't believe they took your family's land that dates back nearly a hundred and fifty years."

Hearing all this reminds me of the unfairness of it all. Clearly, I've become more invested in this land loss than I anticipated. Mother Rita must have gotten to me.

"That's the thing, Darius. I always thought we were just plain old regular Lovejoys, but it turns out my family was, like, extraordinary." I've told him about the land, but I left out the story of the Kingdom of the Happy Land. I don't know why I hide it, maybe because I don't want him to think my family is a bunch of cuckoo birds.

"Of course you are. How could you ever think different?"

I shrug off his compliment. Darius always did believe in me.

"Your daddy used to say if there's one thing they aren't making more of, it's land. Precious land."

I'm touched that he remembers something Daddy used to say. I'd forgotten about that. Daddy's people were from rural Maryland, so he knew something about Black families' connection to the earth.

"Hey, you really should open yourself up more. It doesn't hurt to have a cry now and then," he whispers.

"You know I'm not too good at that."

"Tell me about it." He gives me a moment. "So now you're trying to figure out how to hold on to it, even after she's gone?"

"That's what she wants."

"Is it what you want? Because if what you're saying to me is true, it sounds like she doesn't want you or your mother to ever sell it."

"I guess. I'm not really thinking about myself at the moment. I'm just thinking of her."

"Maybe you should start thinking about yourself. You've spent your whole adult life being a mom and following wherever the wind took you. I don't think you ever had a chance to ask yourself what Nikki wants. Maybe it's time."

His words shake me up a little and I bristle. "You didn't seem to mind me following the wind when we were married."

"Nikki, chill. I'm just trying to help."

I'm so on edge right now. Darius should probably just get up and walk away, but he stays.

"I think there's only one answer here," he says. "You've got to buy the land back."

I squint at him. "No. I'm not doing that, and besides, with what money? I don't have much savings outside of my retirement account, and I'm not dipping into that."

"Baby, you don't have a choice." He speaks to me like he used to, and his tenderness finally reaches me. Now tears are filling my eyes. He hands me a tissue from the box on my desk. "Your mama's house is worth a lot more than what she paid for it. Y'all should take out a home equity loan and purchase as many acres as

247

you can afford. You say your grandmother is only using about four acres? Buy those back."

His voice sounds as if it's coming from the bottom of a well. In my head, I calculate the numbers, the interest rate, the taxes and transactional fees. This is the decision I've dreaded ever since Al Thomas suggested it. Now Darius has just confirmed my lack of choices.

I pick up the phone to call my clients. I'm going to convince them to drop their price so I can get a contract on their house. After I call my clients, I'm going to call Mama.

Darius puts the chair back at the empty desk. I mouth *thank you*, and he squeezes my shoulder. He may not be my husband anymore, but I'm glad he's still my friend.

I USE MY travel voucher to book flights to Asheville for both me and Shawnie. She'll visit for just the hearing, but I've made my own return ticket for seven days after arrival. I've already texted Bryan to handle the scheduling with R.J. He responded immediately, and I'm unsettled by how good it felt when he did. I call Mama, but she doesn't answer.

I leave a voicemail: *Mama, I'm going down to North Carolina this weekend for the hearing and taking Shawnie with me. I'll call you once I know something. Love you. Bye.*

Later that night, I'm home alone sitting on my sofa and thinking of all that has happened. I'd been rushing to get back home, but now that I'm home I can't stop thinking about the kingdom. I open my laptop and search the same genealogical website I visited when I was at the library. I use Mother Rita's library card number to access the Hendersonville library databases. I enter my mama's maiden name—"Lorelle Lovejoy"—and her birthplace—"Hendersonville, North Carolina." It returns over eight thousand results. I've never used one of these sites before, so I'm shocked at the number. Surely there aren't that many Lorelle Lovejoys.

I return to the previous window and check the box marked "Exact" for the names entry. This time I get just a few results, such as Mama's high school yearbook photos. One of those directory listings leads me to Mother Rita. From there, I find my granddaddy Herbert's obituary as well as his draft card and their marriage certificate.

I go back and narrow the search to census records. Mother Rita was born in 1944, so I search the 1950 census. I find their household and enlarge the screen so I can read.

My great-grandmother Lily. When I click on Lily's name, her death certificate pops up.

NAME: Lily Lovejoy
SEX: Female
COLOR OR RACE: Negro
DATE OF BIRTH: 12-21-1908
DATE OF DEATH: 04-10-1980
STATE OF BIRTH: North Carolina
AGE: 72
OCCUPATION: Teacher
PLACE OF DEATH: Henderson County, N.C.
FATHER'S NAME: Vernon Lovejoy
MOTHER'S NAME: Cordelia Montgomery Lovejoy
DEATH CAUSED BY: Probable cardiac standstill; died in sleep

Lily had been a teacher, a Bennett College graduate. I cannot help but swell with pride. I wonder where she taught and if the school still stands. Cordelia. Lily's mother was Cordelia. The discovery of these facts about my family roots me to the chair. I sit back and fold my arms, my head rushing with questions. It hasn't just been my grandmother I've been missing. It has been all of my people. As my mother's only child, I've never even had a sibling to study. Every time I look through these records I feel different, as if I'm finally able to consider my hands, arms, and elbows, belonging to other women.

Whose voice infuses mine? Whose calves shape mine? The same eerie feeling I got while standing in the old kingdom palace washes over me.

And the names. Cordelia. Lily. Rita. What must it have meant to not only lay claim to one's own family but to name one's babies, to answer the census taker's questions as a way of permanency— so different from the white man's property ledger, where he named you what he wanted, excluded a last name, identified you by a scar, and guessed your age. Had I known all this, I might have named my daughter after one of these women.

The idea of an African kingdom in the United States had seemed laughable to me at first. Impossible. Surely the law or Klan or some jealous types would have broken it up. But not only am I now a believer, I am a product of that story. Living and breathing proof that they existed.

I glance at the clock—9:07 p.m. I shake my head to clear it, pick up my cell phone, and press Mother Rita's name.

The phone rings and rings, and I am just about to hang up before she answers.

"Hi, Mother Rita, it's me."

"I'm so glad to hear your voice, Veronica," she says. "I miss you already."

THIRTY

Luella

Sunny was seventeen years old, so it should have come as no surprise to me when the young man Vernon asked for her hand. He came to us in the clearing on a Saturday afternoon in the spring of 1895, after the day's tasks had ended. In the seventeen years since the railroad was completed, families had moved out of the kingdom. As the elders had passed on to heaven—Margaret and George, Papa, Hal, and others—some younger ones decided they didn't like being up on the hill so far away from everything.

Some of the remaining kingdomfolk worked at the nearby inns in summer when the vacationing population rose up. Others left to live and work as hired hands on farms. At least three youngsters I'd known since birth went to work at the tannery in Hendersonville and still others at the gristmill. Demand for liniment had slowed, so even the women had to make do. We still grew our own food, sold vegetables. Wherever there was opportunity, we found it. If I can say one thing about the kingdom, we knew how to make a way. Where once we had totaled nearly three hundred people, we was now down to less than sixty. And I was now the sole leader of the council, as William never resumed his role after Robert left.

Queen Luella was finally more than a title.

William sat next to me, drinking from a cup, a blanket over his legs because he was known to catch a chill even on warm days. I used a needle and thread to close a hole in one of Wade's socks.

As Sunny and Vernon neared us, I carefully placed the sock down in my lap and rearranged my skirt. "Here come Sunny and Vernon," I signaled their arrival to William.

I could tell something was different. Vernon was wearing his Sunday best even though it was Saturday. He held tightly to Sunny's hand as the two of them made a straight line for us. I knew right then and there in my heart I was about to lose my only girl.

The taller Sunny grew, the more I'd worried she wouldn't find a husband. I'd never forgotten when Robert told me that in his daddy's village, some women leaned down to kiss the men. And so when she brought Vernon home, I wondered if Robert's words had been prophecy. The man was a full head shorter than my long-legged girl.

Vernon may not have stood as tall as the Montgomery brothers, but he was as mirthful as Robert and as intelligent as William. And I had noticed on more than one occasion that he made my girl laugh. The young man was slow to anger, even when Sunny did the kinds of things that made me want to sigh—like when she left the window open and it rained inside the house all day or when she forgot to tighten Delight's rope and the mule wandered off and was lost for two days—Vernon just laughed and teased her. He viewed her forgetfulness as charm, her spirited tongue as a challenge, her sass as seduction. I'd met his father once, and the man was the same.

So when the two of them walked up that hill, Sunny towering over him, my heart was eased by the knowledge that I was losing my girl to a man who could make her smile and didn't mind standing on his toes.

"Mr. Montgomery. Queen Luella." He removed his hat.

William sat up straight and picked up his stick, placing a hand atop its chiseled end.

"Please sit." I pointed to two flat rocks near us. When the weather permitted, we spent as much time as we could outside. Over the years, we'd become true mountain people, gathering rocks for propping our feet, using nature's gifts as chairs.

"I suppose what I'm about to say won't come as no surprise."

William nodded ever so slightly.

"I got steady work down at the foundry."

"That's better than the mines," William said. The mines continued to hire our men, and though the pay was fair, sickness and injuries was still common, even with the electric lights they had now.

"Yes, sir, it is." He glanced over at Sunny, who was looking off into the distance as she waited for him to finish his speech. "I want to marry Sunny in my church," Vernon declared. He hadn't actually asked for her hand yet, so the sudden mention of a church startled me.

"We got married here in the kingdom"—I waved my arm—"right over in that clearing. What's wrong with getting married here on the mountain? It's as holy as any church. Papa saw to that."

"Ma, I want to have a fine wedding." Sunny finally turned to look at me. "They say they will do a nice meal in the fellowship hall, too."

"Where will you live?" William asked this question, but with the mention of a church wedding, it was already written on the wall that the two didn't plan to live in the kingdom. I'd always held out hope Sunny would move into one of the empty houses and make her family.

"We plan to live with my ma and pa for a while. Then we get our own place."

"But why, when we got empty houses here?" I asked.

He seemed earnest enough, and though I thought he made a fine suitor, it bothered me that he didn't want to live here. More than likely I'd have to walk for half a day just to go see my own daughter. The kingdom couldn't lose all these young people and expect to survive. Without the people, it was just wilderness.

I wanted to ask William to talk to him, but one look in his eye and I could see Vernon wanted no part of the kingdom. He didn't even look out over the land when I pointed, just patiently explained what he wanted. These young folk was all about their own selves, always talking about what they wanted rather than doing what was right for the people. I suppose I'd spoiled my own, but seemed like to me they was all afflicted with this way of thinking.

"If it's alright with your mother, it's fine by me," William said.

I turned to him. He wasn't supposed to admit defeat so easily. And he knew I couldn't deny Sunny nothing. So I just said, "I'll make your dress."

I gave Sunny a hard look. She knew how much I hated sewing, but the last thing I was going to accept was Vernon's mama getting some ideas about the dress.

SUNNY HELPED ME clean up the plates that evening. My daughter was a headstrong girl, but she had a kind streak, her stubbornness born out of love. When somebody was in trouble, Sunny moved heaven and earth. She was a fierce woman with a soft hand. Fiercer than me even. She would make a fine wife.

"I'm going to miss you," I said, wiping a plate.

"Ma, you act like I'm moving to Charleston."

"Charleston! You better not."

Upstairs, we could hear William dragging his bad leg behind him as he moved between rooms.

"A church wedding, huh."

She wiped her forehead with an arm. "You think Daddy'll hear about it and come?"

Robert had left the kingdom ten years ago. At first, he lived in Flat Rock working at an inn. When the season ended, word was that he moved back down to South Carolina. Wade talked about finding his daddy one day, but Sunny had no interest. She always thought he ought to come see her, that it wasn't right for a girl to go out of her way to seek out her own daddy. I stayed quiet about it, but I agreed. I held the same stubborn view that if Robert wanted me back, he would need to walk his behind up that hill and ask. *Beg.* But I'd long ago stopped hoping for that day to come.

"William will stand with you."

"I know he will," she said.

I stacked the plates and dropped two mugs into the dirty pail of water. Each year, this rift had grown wider and there wasn't nothing I could do about it. Rather than make William leave, he'd just stayed, raising and enjoying the children as if they was his own. And he'd gladly stood by my side and supported my leadership as I had once done for him. For as long as the kingdom had been in existence, the Montgomery family had been at the center of it. Folks politely didn't mention the fact that my children wasn't William's, or that I'd spent nearly ten years with Robert living as husband and wife.

It had been heartbreak for me after I lost my papa. And Robert never even came back to see about me. Some things was unforgivable. The man was my children's daddy, but that was it as far as I was concerned. It was a shame, but it was just the way things had worked out. At least, that's what I told myself.

"When you planning to make it official?"

"Vernon say he got to get a little more money together. He don't want us living with his family too long. He want us to get our own place."

"So y'all going to be out there living on a white man's property."

"Who say it's got to be a white man's property? There is coloreds that rent out houses. Maybe we live in one of theirs."

"Hmm."

Sunny wrapped her arms around me from behind. "I know what you thinking, Ma. You ain't losing me. I won't never go far from here, and I'll be back so much you going to wonder if I'm even married. These hills always be where my heart is."

I placed a hand against hers. "You say that now, but once you have babies of your own it won't be that easy."

"I already know how to tie a baby to my back. And I got two legs, don't I."

"Oh, sure you do." I slapped her thigh with the rag and she giggled. Knowing Sunny, I could just see her with one baby tied to the front and the other to the back, trudging up that hill. The thought pleased me.

At that moment, I determined in my head that I would do everything I could to make sure Robert was at that church wedding for Sunny.

First, I'd have to find him.

———

AIN'T NO EASY way to put it other than to tell it like it was. After Robert moved out, William moved into my bed. It wasn't something we discussed. Wade was growing up, and he wanted his room back. William was having trouble climbing the stairs. My bed was empty.

I was aware that at any time I could've asked William to move and find another place. There was nobody forcing him to share my bed. But it just felt comfortable to me, and I knew it felt comfortable to him, too. He was my friend, and on my loneliest nights, he was a comfort. We hadn't been together long as a married couple, but Papa had raised me to honor vows, and them lessons was hard to unlearn. Once I forgave William, bringing him back was easy since he was still my legal husband.

I did wonder if somehow Robert had heard that me and William slept together now, if the reason Robert didn't return was that he suspected me and William was sleeping together in a way that was like husband and wife. Though we wrapped each other with our arms at night, we never did more than that. Sometime along the way, William had lost his ability to be aroused. He was too proud to ever tell me that outright, but I suspected it. We was family, more than brother and sister but less than husband and wife. It was hard to explain, so I didn't. But I'd be lying if I didn't admit to myself that I ached inside, that I'd been hurting ever since Robert walked out that door.

One night in late spring, a few weeks after we gave Vernon Lovejoy permission to marry Sunny, I pulled on my gown and waited for William to come to bed. He sat on the side of the bed and pulled off a sock.

"Vernon seem like he going to make her happy, don't you think?" I began.

"I believe so," he said. "But I sure wish they'd live here in the kingdom. We could put him on the council."

"We did a good job growing up the young people. They can all read, figure. But we can't make them stay," I said.

"You sure right about that."

I deliberated my words as he pulled off his other sock. Should I tell him that Sunny wanted Robert at the wedding? I didn't want to hurt him, and I knew he loved Sunny as if she was his own. So I put it on myself. "I think Robert ought to give Sunny over to Vernon at the wedding."

"Make sense."

"He is her daddy, after all." I bit my lip.

"Never said he wasn't."

"I don't know if he'll come. I don't even know how to get word to him."

"I'm sure the men'll know. We can send Wade and one of the boys."

"I suppose Robert still work up here in summertime. He might be here already."

"That's possible."

"You seen him?"

"I'd tell you if I had," he said.

I placed a hand on William's back. "I know this ain't easy for you, William. I know how much you love your family."

I felt him relax beneath my touch.

"I accepted this house a long time ago," he said.

It wasn't easy to raise another man's children, especially when those children belonged to your wife and your brother. I had tried to smooth things, but some things was impossible to overcome.

"Sunny going to make a pretty bride. I got to find some nice fabric for the dress."

"Yes, she will." He swung his legs onto the bed. It sank beneath his weight.

"How about we celebrate, just me and you? Take a walk in the morning and listen to the birds the way we used to?"

He turned to me and tucked an arm around my middle. "Got to get up early if we going to catch the baby birds."

"I got some seed we can give them."

He began to whistle softly. "Remember when I could whistle all their songs? I used to be so good at that."

"I do remember that. You was like a bird daddy."

We both laughed, and I turned to snuff out the candle.

"William?"

"Hmm?"

"Speaking of daddies, you my children daddy, too. I just want you to know that. They even got your blood."

"I know that, Luella." He patted my hand and, in the darkness, I could feel him smile.

THIRTY-ONE

I was determined to make Sunny the finest wedding dress the
kingdom had ever seen. We had never called her a princess, but
in my mind, she deserved a dress that fit the position. I went to
find Jola first. My friend had never married, always insisting she
preferred her own company, and I didn't doubt her. She still lived
in the same cabin she'd shared with her parents before they went
to heaven. Her brother and his family lived in the cabin right
across from hers. The kingdom numbers might have been getting
smaller, but it was a good place for a woman without a husband.
Jola offered to help me with Sunny's dress but warned she didn't
have long to work because she was planning to go down to the
coast for a visit with her cousin.

I told Jola to go on her trip and don't worry about the dress.
She suggested a woman in town who could sew the tail off a pea-
cock if you gave her a needle and thread. I took Sunny to the
woman's house for measurements, and with one long sweep of a
look that ended at Sunny's feet, she told us, *You going need plenty*

fabric. I wanted Sunny to have a dress on the ground at her feet, which the lady told me was called a train. I responded I didn't understand why they called it a train and not a tail. She responded that tails was for men.

I wanted to put some lace on her head, but Sunny said *That's enough, Ma* and settled it. This was my only daughter and I had a feeling Vernon would stick with her until one of them was dead in the ground. He wasn't like the Montgomery brothers with all their mess. My girl had picked a simple man, the best kind. I went back to Jola and asked if, on second thought, she could bring the fabric back from Charleston.

Vernon's people belonged to a church called Mud Creek Missionary Baptist Church in Flat Rock, and the wedding would be held there. His father was part of a group of local blacksmiths who was well respected in town. There was no tension between the kingdomfolk and the townsfolk, but we was different. A lot of Flat Rock coloreds had come up from Charleston, working in the summer inns. They was seasonal, some of them traveling back south after summer ended, while others made a home in North Carolina.

On the mountain, most days the women dressed plain. We wore shawls to keep our shoulders warm. Hats to block the sun. Shoes made for walking. That's not to say we didn't pretty up on occasion. A Sunday dress was something special, a Sunday hat a treasure. And we took our time styling our hair in ways that flattered.

No, we was not going to that church house to have people wonder what kind of crazy people called themselves royalty and couldn't even put the princess in a proper wedding dress. We was going to show them that the kingdom was far from ragtag.

We was African royalty.

———

ALL SUMMER, THE lady in town worked on Sunny's wedding dress. To make more money and buy some ribbon for my girl, I started to sell bunches of my flowers. I didn't know why anybody would buy flowers, flowers they could have grown in their own yards, but they loved mines especially after I put them in glass jars. They especially loved my roses, which grew so pretty on the mountain. Some of the white women was so taken by my jars of flowers, they asked me to bring them every week. Their house servants met me at the back door, and I delivered. Sometimes I peered through their windows so I could see my jars setting on gleaming wood tables.

I still worried the Lovejoys would be embarrassed by us, so I decided to do something extra special to show them who we was. One day, while riding the cart with Jola to a woman's house to deliver flowers, I shared an idea.

"I know what we do," I told my friend.

"I didn't know we was doing something."

"We going to fill that church with roses."

"What church?"

"The church where Sunny and Vernon going to marry. Mud Creek."

"Oh, I see." She smacked her thigh. "Girl, you something! Between the roses, Sunny's dress, and the robes we making for you and William, they are going learn about the kingdom!"

We both laughed. The locals didn't blink twice when news spread that Vernon was marrying Sunny. But nobody was marching up the hill trying to live in our community anymore. The years had long passed when Reverend Couch went out in search of new residents. And now it was as if the whole town was waiting for the news when the kingdom would be a bedtime story, just like the stories about the land over the sea where we was stolen.

The vision of that plain little church filled with flowers rose up before my eyes. Sunny didn't want an outdoor wedding, so I would bring the outdoors inside. We would surround the young couple with God's bounty, and when they walked out as a married pair we would throw petals at their feet.

ON THE MORNING of the wedding, I woke up early to take the roses to the church. Me and Jola framed the doorway with blooms and tied stems around the cupola at the altar. We draped the church windows with stems and placed six sprays of flowers at the front of the church. A sweetness filled the sanctuary, and as I stepped back and admired what we'd done, I knew Sunny would love it.

When it was time to get dressed, Wade helped William into the frock coat the Widow had gifted him all them years ago. I wore an old dress turned new again with velvet ribbon sewn the length of the bodice. I'd trimmed my hat in the same ribbon and tucked in a fresh rose blossom along the brim. Once we was ready, we hitched the wagon to Delight, and I took Sunny aside. "You ready to be a married woman?"

"I can hardly breathe. Is this how you felt when you married Uncle William?"

I paused, unsure how to answer. My children knew me and Robert hadn't been married before God, and in truth, that was the time I had felt like she was feeling right now.

"William was the most dignified man I had ever seen," I answered truthfully.

"How did you know you was ready?" She arranged her dress.

"In them days, getting married meant you was a woman. I was ready to leave my papa's house."

"That's more than I can say. I ain't sure I'm ready to be a woman. I just want to be with Vernon."

I pulled the end of her long gown to my chest so that the ground would not soil it. My Sunny was nearly eighteen years old, and though I knew this was a natural time to marry, I still thought of her as a child. "You know something I learned? We don't have too much choice when life come calling. God sent you a good man. God knew it was time and that's what matter most."

"But what it mean to be a woman, Ma?"

The ring of William's and Wade's laughter trickled out to us.

"It mean when it come time to make a decision, you step right up to it. It mean when life send you hardship, you go to bed and get up the next morning to face it."

"And if I don't?"

"Then you leave it to God."

The *tap-tap* of William's stick sounded as he walked down the porch stairs. It was time for us to go, my last moment to speak alone with my daughter over and done with.

Delight had always been more pet than worker, but she would do anything I asked of her. Despite her age, her freshly bathed coat shone in the light. We filled four carts with kingdomfolk. Women rode on the carts to keep their Sunday dresses clean. Men walked alongside us. Not everybody from the kingdom was going to the wedding. We never left our settlement completely un-guarded. A few was too infirm for the trip. In total, a little over forty of us made out for the church.

Since we carried the bride, our wagon was the last in the procession. Sunny sat between me and William. We rode past the Widow's inn, and I thought of how the son was faring after the death of his mother a few years earlier. No wife or children, he spent most of his days just sitting out on his porch reading them poetry books he'd always loved. That old lady had been nice to us and probably would've sent a wedding gift on Sunny's special day. He waved from the porch, and some of the men waved back.

At the church, Wade helped us out of the wagon. Somebody inside was playing the piano, and the plink of keys filled the air. Dust swirled as the carts pulled to a stop and the kingdom people descended. By the sound of it, Vernon's people was already inside. We would all march in and take our seats before the bridal march started up. That was how we'd planned it.

"How y'all doing?" Wade said to a group of women walking up. At almost fifteen years old, tall for his age, he was a charmer.

William waited patiently for me to take his arm, leaning ever so slightly on his stick.

"Hey there, Lu."

I knew that voice anywhere and, at first, I didn't respond. Finally, I turned around and saw Robert walking up. I almost cried out. I hadn't seen him in years. He had gained a few pounds, and he was filling out his suit. Somehow I kept my feelings close, the storm of them.

"You made it!" Sunny didn't hold back her excitement. We was lucky the children didn't still blame either one of us for what happened. In the early years, they swung from confusion to anger and back again. These days they accepted our situation, mostly because they was so fond of William. They'd grown to love their uncle, and if they could've had both men living in the same house again, they would have.

"I wouldn't miss my baby girl's wedding for all the money in the U.S. government bank," Robert declared as he kissed her on the cheek. I frowned at him, wondering how such words could drip off his tongue. He had missed plenty in his girl's life, and his boy's, too. But it wasn't the moment to have that conversation.

"Brother," William said.

"Brother," Robert replied.

"What he look like these days, Luella?"

I tried to choose the right words. "He look like he ready to go in a church for a wedding. We see y'all in the church."

I turned to give Sunny one more squeeze, but her eyes was drowning in her daddy's. Even Wade was hanging around looking at him instead of helping the elders inside.

William pushed his arm against my side so I could grab hold of it. "I'm glad he showed up," he whispered.

When we walked into the church, all the kingdomfolk was on one side and Lovejoys on the other. The perfume of the roses was even stronger than it had been in the morning, as the blooms opened up in the heat. I could feel the Lovejoys staring at me and William, so I turned and nodded. Soon Vernon's family would be ours. And our people would be his people. I caught his mother's eyes as she smiled. A nice lady. I'd met her twice. The Lovejoys may have insisted on us coming to their church, but we had contributed our portion.

Once me and William was up front and the last few guests, including Wade, had taken their seats, the bridal march began and everybody stood. I turned to see my Sunny marching beside Robert, step by step. Finally, I understood what he had meant about the stories of tall women in Africa, the respect they'd been given, their majesty. My daughter had never looked so beautiful. She wasn't a princess no longer. She was going to be the queen of her own household. The head of her own Lovejoy line.

When they was up at the front of the church, the minister said in a loud, booming voice, "Who gives this bride?" And Robert answered proudly, "I do." I half expected William to speak up at the same time as Robert in answer to that question. He wouldn't have been wrong if he had. Vernon took Sunny's arm, and Robert took his seat at the other end of the row. I glanced down and noticed a woman seated beside him. She patted his hand, and I blinked twice slowly.

Robert must have married. And he had brought his new wife to the wedding and paraded her right in front of me.

THIRTY-TWO

During the whole entire wedding and the meal after, I tried to avoid Robert and his new woman, and when he dared look my way, I turned the other direction. After all the festivities ended, on the way back up the hill, William said to me, "They say Robert brought a woman with him. I wonder who is she. I suppose it wouldn't be no surprise that after being gone all these years, he moved on."

"Yes, but bring her here? In front of everybody in the kingdom?" I hissed.

William said nothing, and I knew we shouldn't discuss it no longer.

The next morning, I went outside to dig up bulbs and replant them. The worst thing about winter was not having my flowers, but this would be my first winter without Sunny. I spread out a sackcloth and kneeled on it, turning to look up at the sky. It was still early, but the sun beat down on my face hard enough to make me squint. I couldn't stop thinking about Robert's woman, how kind and pleasant she'd been at the wedding. I'd even seen her hug Sunny. The nerve of some people. I held up my hands, turned them over to the back. I had never been the kind of woman who took much pleasure in my looks, but I'd been considered a beauty in my young days and it was hard to let go of that kind of power.

Seeing Robert after all these years had stirred up my old feelings. I thought I'd been over him, but the sight of that woman and the burn in my chest told something different.

"Lu."

I turned, startled. There Robert stood, hat in hand, the woman beside him, William hovering behind them. He wasn't wearing the fancy suit he'd worn to the wedding, just a pair of regular work pants. It was the Robert of old, except his hair had started to pull back from his face.

"What you doing up here?" I asked, nervous all of a sudden.

"I came to introduce you to Ursula."

"Introduce me to who?" I wiped my hands on my skirt as I stood up. The woman standing beside him watched me eagerly. She was wearing a hat that shielded her face and a locket on a chain around her neck. I couldn't stop staring at the locket. Was Robert's picture inside? The force of my jealousy surprised me.

"I've heard a lot about you," she said.

I looked from her to Robert. I even glanced behind them at William, who was smiling ear to ear like a fool. What was his problem?

"I'm sorry I can't say the same," I said, looking at Robert. I didn't know whether to feel humiliated or honored.

"This is our sister Ursula. She was sold away from our mama when she was a little girl. I been looking for her, and I finally found her down in Charleston. She wanted to come with me to Sunny's wedding, but we didn't want to disrupt things with a big old reunion."

"Your sister?"

"We ain't seen her since she was a little girl," William called out. "I still can't believe it. Last time I saw Ursula, she was wearing pigtails!"

"Your sister?" I said again. She wasn't tall like the brothers, but now that I looked closely, the face was the same as William's.

"When I left here, I went searching for some of our family. I thought I'd come back after I got my head right. But there was so many of us sold off by the Montgomerys. I found four brothers and sisters in the first two years."

Ursula nodded at me, as if affirming Robert's accounting of his whereabouts.

"Once I started finding them, I couldn't stop. I know I owe you more than that, and God knows I owe my children. But Luella, I found ten of my brothers and sisters. Ten." His voice broke, and Ursula put an arm around his shoulder.

"William, you didn't know that was your own sister at the wedding?" I yelled loud enough for him to hear. I knew I sounded foolish, but I didn't know what else to say in my embarrassment.

William didn't spare me. "I thought she was Robert's woman, same as you."

Robert laughed. "Luella Montgomery, you thought I had married again?"

"Come on, William." Ursula backed up and took the older brother's arm. "Let's go back to the house so I can hear more about the kingdom. Robert said you the man to ask."

Robert put his chin to his chest, then sat down on the sackcloth, motioning for me to do the same. We was so far away from the palace he could've placed his head in my lap and his brother and sister wouldn't have seen. I found myself wishing he would. I knew I should be mad at him, but I couldn't help my feelings. My desire for him had not waned one bit.

"How did you find them?" I remembered how upset he'd been that him and William was fighting over me, how he'd called him the only family he had left, how they called each other *brother* as if it was a sacred word.

"A lot of us still out there searching for our kin. I know it ain't no excuse, but we came from a place down on that plantation where love ties was thin as air, where children went to sleep alongside us and was disappeared by morning."

I froze. "Robert."

"We got to open this thing up, Lu. We can't keep putting it away forever."

I grabbed his hand and squeezed it hard. If he started opening up about the past, about the things we'd seen, we would both have to do it and it might kill a little piece of us all over again. "Is this an apology? If so, ain't no need."

"I know you heard about how they sold the little ones. It was all true. Me and my brother was kept around as their most valued. But so many was sold. So many, Lu. When it was all over, my ma had born nineteen babies." His voice broke.

"Hush, Robert. I don't want to hear it." I placed a hand on his leg.

"Them little children they sold was our brothers and sisters, Luella. That's why I been searching, trying to find some of them. And now I got a sister that I barely even remember." He began to cry.

"What's done is done." I clenched my heart shut, afraid of what his tears might open up in me. "Look how far we've come."

I didn't know what to say to him. It felt like enough for for-
giveness, but it couldn't wash away my years of hurt. I had cried so
many tears over this man, what we could have had, what we lost.
But I couldn't blame him for what slavery did to us, how it messed
us up on the insides so that love became something more complicated than it was ever meant to be.

"So do you got a new woman or not?"

"Lu."

I was a child again. Petulant. Insufferable.

"There ain't but one woman for me." He reached for my chin
and touched it gently with a finger.

"I was your woman, once."

"No, you was my wife."

"That's not what my papa said."

"That's why you couldn't make up your mind? Your papa told
you William was still your husband?"

"Papa dead."

"I hurt when we lost him, too."

"Is that why you up and left?"

"I left because I didn't want to be your second husband. I
needed a woman who could give me all of her."

"I tried."

"Your lips said one thing but my eyes saw another."

"A woman need time to settle things."

"And now?"

"And now what?" I turned to him. He was only inches from
me, but it was as if he was miles away. I wanted to be closer to
him, and then closer some more, to smell his neck and see if the
little hairs on his chin still scratched.

"How long does a woman need now?"

"What you mean?"

"I mean"—he cleared his throat—"I mean, if I was to come back, how long would you need to settle things?"

I closed my eyes, too afraid to give in to this hope after all my heartbreak.

"Not even a day," I whispered finally, looking at him.

ROBERT NEEDED MORE time to settle things on his end, so he traveled back to South Carolina with Ursula. He had promised her husband he would safely return her to Charleston. The days that followed his departure was tough. Part of me wondered if he would return at all. Maybe it was all in my imagination.

Both of us had sat down with William, paid him the respect of asking for his blessing once again. At first I was afraid William wouldn't understand, that he'd ask me to stay. But he seemed resigned to it, and in the days after we spoke, I understood that William had held another emotion all these years. Guilt. He had broken up his brother's family, and once the damage had been done, he had not wanted to leave us in bits and pieces. So he'd stayed and tried to make the best of things.

Now it was time for William to move on and he knew it. On the day of his move to Papa's empty cabin, I helped him pack his things.

"I left the cape in the closet," he said, standing in the doorway of our bedroom.

"The king's cape?"

"I ain't been king in a long time."

"Stop talking nonsense. It belongs to you."

"No." He shook his head. "You the one and true ruler, Luella. You should wear it."

It was true. I had been leading the council ever since Robert's departure. I kept the ledger containing our treasury notes. I had brought more women onto the council, including Jola. The women now had equal say. Today folks came to me with their problems, men and women alike.

I didn't know how to put into words what William meant to me. Maybe there wasn't even words for it. We sat down together on the bed. All them years ago, when he'd struck me across my face, was ancient history. Now he was just this gentle man who had led us here, helped us build a life away from the Klan and the threats down in South Carolina, and who was humble enough to follow me as queen after I became the chosen leader.

"I bet you wish you never got mixed up with the Montgomery brothers," he said.

"How could I wish that?"

"You ain't deserve two men leaving you, let alone two brothers. We ain't done right by you the way we should have."

"You done more than most."

He stood, but I wouldn't let go of his hand, so I stood with him. "You want to walk with me and listen to the birds?"

"Alright, Luella," he said. "Let's walk."

TWO WEEKS PASSED and Robert was still not back from Charleston. Both Wade and I waited as if we was waiting for the president of the United States. We cleaned the house and chopped wood to get ready for winter. It was pickling season, but instead of helping the women, I swept the yard, washed the bedclothes, cleaned house, all while keeping one eye on the lane. A part of me feared Robert wouldn't keep his word, but I just couldn't believe he would do this to me twice. I wanted to send a message to him that William had moved out of the palace, but Wade told me not to waste money on a telegram.

So I waited.

Wade occupied his time with a young woman, and I knew that sometimes they snuck off. There was no stopping a fifteen-year-old boy from smelling himself, so I spent a lot of time alone in the house, missing Sunny. She hadn't visited since the wedding, and once I thought she'd had enough time to be a new wife, I planned to walk and pay her a visit.

The day I sent word to Sunny I was coming to visit, the sound of a drumhead rang through the air. We had built a small house at the gate, and one of the widowers had lived there for close to six years. I couldn't remember the last time he'd hit that drum. The sound could only mean one thing: trouble. I could hear the kingdom rustling as I walked out onto my porch. I couldn't help but think of that time Robert was returned to me beaten by the law. We had paid that debt off years ago when the local sheriff passed on. Besides, we didn't have no money to spare these days. My whole chest stiffened in dread.

Wade walked up behind me. "Who you think it is?"

I shook my head. It would take them a few minutes to climb the hill.

"I'm going to walk down there and see," Wade said.

"Stay right here, son." The palace was back off the main kingdom path. Somebody would come tell me the business soon enough.

I sat down in a chair on the porch and crossed my feet. After a while, I heard the sound of men approaching. When they rounded the corner, William was in the lead, his arm held by

275

Harry. Behind him walked two white men wearing sheriff's badges that glinted in the sun. Wade walked out onto the porch.

"Luella," William called out my name in a high-pitched voice. And he left off the queen. Something was wrong.

I stood and leaned on the railing. "Gentleman, to what do we owe the pleasure of your visit?" My voice was heavy with foreboding.

One of the men removed his hat. His head was bald and mottled with spots. He had a soft chin that folded into his neck. The other man kept his hat on. He was much younger and chewed on a wad of tobacco, his mouth moving quickly like a rabbit. "Ma'am, is that your son, Wade Montgomery?"

I stepped in front of Wade, who had stiffened.

"Yes, sir."

"We come to take him with us."

"Why?"

"Luella, we going to follow them into town. Don't worry none. We figure this out right away," William said. He was surrounded by what appeared to be every man in our kingdom. The sheriff and his deputy looked around uneasily, one of them fingering the gun in his holster.

"There was some trouble over in Saluda last night."

"Trouble?"

Saluda was nearly ten miles away.

"Oh, nothing much. Just somebody let out somebody's cows, and we want to find out if your boy the one done it."

"I can tell you right now he ain't the one. Why in the world would he be all the way over there?" Wade had been going out late to see that girl, who I'd heard was a few years older. I wondered if she lived in Saluda. Truthfully, I didn't know where he had been the night before. But I knew my son. He wouldn't have let no-body's cows out of a gate, especially not the cows of a white man. He knew better.

"Somebody saw a colored boy let those cows out. They say it was a boy from the kingdom, and they say it was the queen's son. We just going to take him for a little while to see if this the same boy they seen."

"Last night, you say?"

"Yes, ma'am."

Even without turning to Wade, I knew there was a lie buried in the sheriff's story. At night, nobody could've gotten close enough to say it was Wade for sure.

"It's a lie, Ma," he whispered from behind.

I turned my head slightly to let him know I heard him.

"Wade, you go on with the deputy. We be right behind you," William called out.

William was trying to tell me we had no choice. But some-thing in my body wouldn't let my only son pass. I couldn't just give my boy over to these men. I might never see him again. I knew what could happen to boys his age, law or no law. We lived here in the kingdom to protect us from this very kind of thing. I never should've let Wade wander off to see that girl. I should've kept him here on the hill, where he was safe.

I shook my head.

"Luella." William stepped forward. "We get it all worked out. I promise."

I shook my head again. The deputy fingered his pistol.

"It's alright, Ma." Wade stepped out from behind me. "Send word to Daddy," he whispered.

At the mention of Robert, I gathered my wits. I put my arm

around Wade. He squeezed me and pulled away. The sheriff's deputy led the way down the hill, followed by a small knot of kingdom men.

Only William stayed behind, standing in the middle of the lane. As soon as they was out of sight, I went to him and grabbed hold of his hand.

Why hadn't Robert come like he said he would?

THIRTY-THREE

Nikki

I magine my surprise when I arrive at Mother Rita's that Sunday
and come upon my mama's car, covered in a layer of dust and
parked in the driveway. I can see how learning that Mother Rita
has cancer convinced her to get down here quickly. Not to mention the prospect of eviction. I'd just never expected that in a
week's time we would all be in this house together.

"Grandma is here?" Shawnie says from the passenger seat beside me. I've filled her in on everything during the plane ride. She
was less shocked than I was about the kingdom, accepting the
story without question. She's even excited to see the old palace.

"She must have driven down here." I don't know what else
to say.

Four generations of Lovejoy women are about to be in the
same room, and I'm not sure I'm prepared for that.

The front door is unlocked, as Mother Rita prefers. A duffel
bag sits in the foyer. The drive from D.C. takes eight hours. Of

course, Mama plans to stay overnight. I assume I'll take the sofa and give her and Shawnie the bedroom.

The air carries the scent of what I've come to recognize as the magic of Mother Rita's navy beans. In the refrigerator there will be a freshly prepared salad. When the beans are almost ready, Mother Rita will unhook the skillet and pour the batter for the skillet bread. I feel the tug of returning to something warm, familiar.

We drop our bags and I lead Shawnie into the kitchen.

It doesn't appear Mama has been here long. She and Mother Rita are sitting across from each other at the table, silent.

"Mama, I didn't know you were coming. You didn't respond to my voicemail or texts."

I can feel Shawnie staring at Mother Rita. Her eyes flick from her to Mama and finally to me. I want to wrap my arms around my daughter, protect her from all the hurt that has such a hold over the lives of the women in our family.

"I decided to come at the last minute," is all Mama says.

Mother Rita rises from her chair. She looks thin, but it has only been two weeks since I left. Her face is stricken, as if she can scarcely believe all four of us are in her kitchen.

"Shawnie." She holds a hand out. "I haven't seen you since you were this high."

Shawnie steps forward cautiously, and Mother Rita wraps her arms around her. Shawnie relaxes, and I watch as my daughter closes her eyes, allowing the affection.

I'd always thought the sight of my mama and Mother Rita in the same room, finally, would make me cry. But it is my daughter and her great-grandmother that does it. My eyes overflow.

"I guess this is a family reunion." I don't even know why I am saying this. Family reunions are supposed to be joyous. This moment is terrifying. With all of us in the room together, there's no place to hide. All the silences, all the little slights that have chipped away at my relationship with Shawnie and at Mama's relationship with Mother Rita are now right out in the open.

Mother Rita claps her hands together. "Now, y'all two go wash up and come sit with us. Lunch will be ready shortly. Shawnie, I hope you like beans."

"Yes, ma'am."

In the bathroom, I show Granddaddy Herbert's photograph to Shawnie. "Wasn't he handsome?" I say.

She doesn't respond. I can only guess how she's feeling, so I don't press her. I'm upset with myself for us not visiting sooner, years sooner. I have taken on the guilt that should only belong to the eldest women in the family. It's fully my own now and regret tightens my chest.

Back in the kitchen, I sit in the fourth chair and look between my mama and Mother Rita, wondering how they'd greeted each other when Mama first showed up at the door. Had Mother Rita hugged her daughter as she did Shawnie? Had Mama been startled by Mother Rita's appearance? Had Mother Rita even known she was coming? My throat is dry and scratchy. I need water, but I don't dare get up.

"I sure was glad to hear from your mama when she called," Mother Rita says to me, her voice jittery with nerves. She has prepared a meal for all of us, a sure sign of her excitement. "It's been too long."

"What time did you get here, Mama?" I ask.

"Just a few minutes before you arrived." Mama's voice is flat.

"Mother Rita, do you want me to set the table for lunch?" asks Shawnie.

"That would be lovely. Plates are in the dining room cabinet, and everything else you need is in those two drawers there."

Shawnie disappears into the dining room, as if aware she needs to give us all a minute.

"Why didn't you tell me you were sick?" Mama asks.

Mother Rita's lips purse. I've been around her sharp tongue enough now to know when harsh words are threatening to slip out. Instead, she somehow manages a soft tone. "If I had told you, would it have made any difference?"

"Of course it would have made a difference."

"She called me," I interrupt. "Isn't that the same?"

They both glance at me, and I realize this is a conversation for the elders. I should probably go and help Shawnie, but I'm too deeply buried in this sandpit of grief.

"Veronica did her best to help."

"You know she prefers Nikki," Mama corrects her.

"Did you ever tell her that I named her? Did you tell her that?"

I turn to Mama. I know Mother Rita is not completely innocent in all this, but the hits just keep coming.

Shawnie comes back into the kitchen and rattles around in the silverware drawer. They wait until she leaves again before they resume speaking, as if she can't hear every word being spoken in this small house.

"You've got her thinking I'm such a bad person," Mama says. "Did you tell her you were the person who said you never wanted to speak to me again? That I was as good as dead to you?"

"You sold me down the river!" Mother Rita cries.

"It wasn't my fault."

Mother Rita lowers her voice and speaks as if from her depths.

"My people did everything to keep this land and you stood by and did nothing while they robbed us."

"It wasn't your rightful land, Mama."

"Who are you to make that decision? You not the law, judge, and jury."

"There was nothing I could do." Mama's voice is soft.

"You didn't even try."

This accusation feels disturbingly familiar, and so does my mama's response to it. I look from one to the other and back again, trying to figure it all out. How had Mama sold Mother Rita out? What was the betrayal that was bad enough to cause eight years of silence?

"You never felt nothing for this land. You left it behind like a can of garbage."

"I know that's how you feel—that I left you and Daddy behind—but I just needed to go out on my own."

Mama is right. Mother Rita is conflating the land and the family. Mother Rita took Mama's departure as personal, rather than as a young woman finding her own way.

"You didn't just leave us, though. You"—Mother Rita points out the window—"treated the loss of the land like it wasn't nothing."

Mama's eyes flash. "What difference does it make if we lose it? None of us is moving back here to this old scrubby mountain, anyhow."

"It makes a whole hell of a difference, Lorelle. It's our legacy! This land made us who we are!"

The kitchen is hot with their breath. In the other room, it's quiet, as if Shawnie has paused her tasks long enough to let the storm pass.

"You mean that old cockamamie story that you could never let go of? Growing up, all you talked about was the kingdom this and the kingdom that. There ain't even proof your queen wore a crown."

Mother Rita shakes her head. I fear she's going to pass out.

"Both of you, please!" I stand and put both hands up. "That's enough. We are all here now and what's past is past. Let's concentrate on the time we have left, and by that I mean today."

Mama opens her mouth to say something, but I raise a finger. "You and I can talk when we get back home. But for now, we are here on this mountain and we are going to be a family."

I walk over to the stove and unhook the skillet. Shawnie comes back in the kitchen and retrieves glasses from the counter, as if on cue.

Mother Rita takes a few deep breaths. Then finally she stands and takes the cornmeal out of the cabinet. Only Mama doesn't move from the table.

We haven't solved all our problems, but for the moment, we will sit together and we will eat.

THIRTY-FOUR

Luella

The lie was bigger than I'd imagined. The kingdom had lulled me to sleep. Surrounded by colored men, the sheriff's deputy had not revealed the real charge against Wade, and I should have known. It was bulls that had been let loose. And a man had been found trampled to death in the pen.

It was the 1890s, and we knew that things was happening to our people. Not just in North Carolina but in places near and far. Men and women hanged from trees. Houses and businesses burned to the ground. Families run off. Lives stolen right out from under us. It was a time when Black folk lived in terror, and we should have known it would come knocking at our doorstep, too, no matter how much we tried to hide away in the hills.

But the kingdom was different, or so we'd believed. They didn't bother us there. We went about our days, working and living and minding our business. White people had liked and bought our liniment. I sold flowers to some of the best families in town. We'd worked hard—supplying food and eggs to the vacationers, working the mines, answering the call from the mills. And when the day was done, we'd returned back to the kingdom, our little piece on top of a hill where we didn't bother nobody and nobody didn't bother us.

Until they came for Wade.

Within a day of them taking our son, Robert arrived in Hendersonville and came straight to me. William had gone to live in Papa's cabin, and I was living alone for the first time in my life. Sunny offered to come stay with me, but all I'd wanted to do was lie in the dark and cry myself to sleep every night. When Robert walked in the door, I was lying in my bed staring at the wall. He came right to me, so swiftly that I barely had time to wonder who was coming in my door without so much as a knock.

I put my head in his lap as he stroked my hair. "It's alright, baby. I'm here. I ain't leaving you no more. I'm here right by your side and we going get our boy home safe."

The next morning we took our time drinking coffee. Robert hadn't taken off his clothes from the day before. I went outside and filled a bowl with fresh water. When I returned, he was sitting in the chair he'd loved when he used to live with us, the same one William had come to occupy every evening after dinner. For a moment, I startled, seeing him back in that chair as if he'd never left it.

I put the bowl of water on the table and lay a cloth next to it.

"Better shave and wash up," I said. "We got to be ready today."

I hadn't slept much, but I was determined that I wasn't lying down in that bed again without my son. I didn't know what I would have to do to get him home. If I couldn't get him out of that jail, I was going to figure out a way for him to run. I'd rather he was on the run from the law for the rest of his days than see his body swing from a tree.

After Robert cleaned up, he told me he'd be right back. I didn't have to ask where he was going. I knew he was going to see his brother. They had no choice but to lean on each other, and I was glad for it. I needed both of the brothers to help Wade through this. Whatever Robert couldn't do, William would. Wade had two daddies, and the three of us would get our boy out of this, even let him marry that girl if he had the mind.

By the time Robert returned, I'd brought Delight around and hitched her to the post next to the palace. The animal kept looking at me, as if she knew something was wrong. I patted her flank, more to calm myself than the old girl.

When we was on our way, Robert turned around to ask me about the lawyer. I'd had such a determined look in my eye that morning, he hadn't even asked me about a plan.

"This is the man done the paperwork when we bought the kingdom," I said.

"You think he fight for Wade?"

"Do we have a choice?"

He didn't have to hurry the mule, who trotted at a naturally brisk pace. The cold fall air stung my cheeks, and I pulled my scarf closer around my head. As we descended the hill, we rounded the bend and the lake. Without my son near me, the air had turned gray with ash, as if we'd reached the end of God's days.

"My brother say there ain't no law in the world that can save him," Robert said after a while. "We need something more than the law."

"What's more than the law?"

He pointed to the sky.

"I'm not going to let them kill my son," I said.

"He say the best we can hope for is a few years in a labor camp."

287

"Camp?" I kept my eyes straight ahead.

"You know that's what they do to us now. Either kill us or work us."

"He ain't but fifteen years on this earth, Robert."

"To them, he a man. You know who laid the railroad?"

"He my boy, and I'm bringing him home."

"If you say so."

"What took you so long to come back?" Until now, I hadn't been able to summon the strength to ask.

"I was with my family."

"We are your family, Robert. Ten years ago, you left me and your children in a night. Now I tell you I'm ready and you off somewhere—"

"I'm here now, Lu. I'm here to stay."

I kept quiet until we reached the small brick building with the plate-glass window. My anger threatened to spill out all over the street. I wanted to smash that window, throw a rock through it and watch it shatter. Across the front was written N. R. WEAVER, ESQ. Briefly, I wondered what the "Esq." meant. In this world, I was all but lost.

Robert held the door for me and asked the lady sitting at the desk if Mr. Weaver was available. The woman put down her pen. She was wearing a plain blouse and her hair was pulled into a bun so tight that the edges of her eyes was pulled back. "Who shall I tell him is asking?"

"My name is Robert Montgomery, and this here my wife, Lu-ella Montgomery. We from the Kingdom of the Happy Land."

She didn't move, as if we was rare birds just landed right smack in front of her. A lot of the town thought us kingdomfolk was strange, if only because we kept to ourselves. Sometimes I wondered what kinds of rumors flowed about us. As long as they didn't say we was up there eating human beings, I didn't pay no mind to the whispers.

"Please have a seat," she said, pointing to the two wooden chairs sitting with their backs against the windows.

Robert motioned for me to sit, but he remained standing, turning sideways so he could keep an eye out the window. But the lawyer kept us waiting so long that I told Robert he ought to sit. He still refused.

Finally, the man who I remembered helping us with the deed to our land came out and said hello. He didn't offer a hand for Robert to shake, but he did invite us back to his office, where he pointed to a seat.

"Mr. and Mrs. Montgomery, I heard about your boy. You must be real shook up about it."

He called us Mr. and Mrs. That gave me courage. I started talking fast, not sure how much time he would allow us, using my fancy voice. "Mr. Montgomery, our boy didn't do the things they say he did. That's why we here. We want to make sure they don't kill him before he go to trial—"

"Make sure who don't kill him?"

Robert put a hand on my arm. "Sir, we just want to make sure he get a fair trial."

"Of course, I understand. I been lawyering in this county a long time. I know justice for your people ain't common."

That statement gave me hope, too. To utter such a thing as a man of the law was not without risk.

Robert continued. "Mr. Weaver, would you help us? I know

you to be a fair man. You helped us out when we bought our land. You go to church every Sunday. You a godly man, and I know that for a fact."

"Why, thank you, Mr. Montgomery. But how can I keep a mob from breaking in that jail and hurting your son? I'd like to help if I could, but—"

So he did know what we meant when we said we hoped *they* wouldn't kill Wade.

"If he do make it to trial," Robert interrupted before the lawyer could say no, "we want you to be his lawyer in court. He ain't but fifteen years old."

"Fifteen?"

"Yes, sir."

"I got a fifteen-year-old grandson. Name is Charlie."

Both me and Robert knew better than to make a comparison between his grandson and Wade, but the lawyer had already done it. So we let that sit with him as he rolled a pencil between his fingers.

"If he do make it to trial, would you be his lawyer? Would you help make sure they don't send him away forever or worse?" I asked pleadingly, whispering the last two words.

"I just don't know."

"Course, we pay you," Robert said.

The lawyer made a little noise in his throat and wrote something on a piece of paper. He passed it to Robert. I glanced over at the number.

Robert looked at me. He had been away from the kingdom for so long that he was surprised to learn that morning we didn't have much money stored away. In the days he'd lived there, we'd had a large treasury. With our dwindling numbers the treasury was much smaller than before. The most valuable thing we owned now was the land.

I grabbed the edge of the desk. "We pay you every month. Like clockwork."

He shook his head. "I don't think that would work out."

"Why not?" I demanded.

"How do I know you're going to pay me back?"

I turned to Robert in a panic. His eyes darted, as if he was trying to figure something else out.

"Because I'm a man of my word and this my son we talking about," said Robert. For a moment, the king appeared. Then I watched as he folded back inside himself.

"I hear you losing a lot of your people up there on the hill. Do y'all still hold the deed to the land?" the lawyer asked.

"Yes, sir," Robert said slowly.

"You still got the paperwork I did for you when you bought it from the Widow Davis?"

"Yes, sir."

"Then that will do," he said.

"What will do?" I repeated.

"You turn over the deed and I'll help your boy."

"You can hold the South Carolina deed. We keep the North Carolina land," I said, wondering if we should have chosen another lawyer who didn't know we held two deeds. We'd hoped we could protect some of it, but Weaver knew everything.

The lawyer looked at Robert, ignoring me, as if refusing to bargain with a woman. "I hold all two hundred five acres and you got a deal."

Robert turned to me. The lawyer was asking too much. We

couldn't give away all our land. It was worth a lot more than the lawyer's fee.

The man rubbed his temples. "But I wonder. Is that land any good, Mr. Montgomery? Ain't most of it just brush? Maybe I'm getting ahead of myself."

Robert recovered quickly. "We got plenty good land. Where you think we grow our food?"

He paused. "Alright. Do we have a deal?"

I wanted to step outside and talk this over with Robert. Even though the deed was in our names, we couldn't make this decision without the council.

But did we have a choice? If we helped Wade escape and he went on the run, they might come to the kingdom and take another person's son. If he stayed in that jail without protection, he might lose his life.

Robert spoke slowly, as if each word cost him. "Alright. But we get it back soon as we save up the money to pay you."

I tried to calm my breath. Robert was William's brother, after all. That was the kind of thing William would have said. There wasn't nothing like an understanding.

"Course. How about I give you two years? If you don't pay me within two years, the deed goes in my name permanently. Puts a date on it."

Robert took a moment, then said, "Alright, then."

"I'll get the paperwork together and send somebody out there to take a look around," he said.

The lawyer stood, and we followed suit. I wasn't going home with my son, but I was going home with something.

"So you won't let them kill our Wade?" I asked.

"Mrs. Montgomery, I will do everything I can to send your boy home to you." He looked me right in the eye when he said it, and I believed him.

We stood to walk out, but just as we was about to leave, I turned back around. Weaver had already sat back down at his desk.

"Thank you, sir," I said.

He didn't look up.

As we climbed in the cart, Robert said to me, "You think he do what he say?"

"He called us Mr. and Mrs. Montgomery. You hear that? He the best we can do," I replied. And that was the truth.

THIRTY-FIVE

I could barely sleep knowing my Wade was sleeping in the jail every night after I left him. When I couldn't get there to sit with him, Sunny visited, and when Sunny couldn't get there, Robert went. Even William made his way down the hill to see about his boy. The women from the kingdom delivered food, because it took time for the judge to say he would hear the case; in the meantime, Mr. Weaver wrote up the papers for our agreement.

All in all, three months passed.

Nobody in the kingdom was too happy with the trade Robert and me made. After the council scolded us for not talking to them first, we reminded them we didn't have a lot of time to come to a decision. They finally agreed under the condition me and Robert alone raised the money to get the deed back. That part of the agreement seemed to put everybody's misgivings at ease, but I worried two years was too short.

Either Mr. Weaver kept his word to help protect my son or my constant prayers caught the wind all the way to God's ear, but

Wade's life was spared during the months he slept in the jailhouse. The dead farmer had owned five acres, and though he wasn't a wealthy man and didn't belong to nobody's church, there was still demand for answers.

The trial began on a Monday morning. The council of elders from the kingdom, which now numbered six not including Robert, sat in the back of the courtroom. They only gave us one row of seats, so we decided it would just be us kingdom leaders and family. I sat next to Sunny. We both wore plain dresses, our hair tied up in scarves. We didn't want to anger the jury for no reason. But when we walked in there, people still whispered and pointed, probably trying to figure out which ones of us was haughty enough to call ourselves royalty.

I hadn't never been in a courtroom before, so I was surprised to see it wasn't no different than a church. At the front of the room Wade sat next to his lawyer. They'd allowed us to bring our son a fresh suit of clothes, but he'd grown thin since arriving in the jail and the clothes hung slack on his body. He kept glancing back at me, and each time he did, I gave him a little smile, trying to send him strength through my eyes.

The jury sat in a box that wasn't no different than a choir stand. The judge in his robe reminded me of a preacher, and the pews was the same hard wooden benches as in churches. Nobody looked our way at the back of the room. It was like we was invisible.

The trial judge said a few things I didn't understand, then announced there would be no opening speeches. He asked a man he called a "prosecutor" to call up his first witness. This man claimed he saw my boy near the victim's property that night "lurking" around. Then the prosecutor called up the farmer's wife, who between a lot of tears claimed she heard her husband shout, as if to scare off somebody, but by the time she ran outside her husband was already gone to be with the Lord. The prosecutor sat, and Mr. Weaver stood to begin his questions. After expressing his condolences, Mr. Weaver asked her: "Have the bulls ever gotten out of the pen before?"

"I don't know, maybe." The wife glanced at the jury and smiled. "Everybody knows that can happen on occasion. But I can't remember the last time it happened."

"But you're saying it's a possibility that the bulls got out on their own and your husband was just the victim of an unfortunate accident?"

"Objection, Your Honor! He's harassing this poor widow!"

"Sustained. Mr. Weaver, I will remind you to be respectful of this court."

"No further questions, Your Honor."

The last witness for the prosecutor was the doctor who told how the bulls ran over the man, how painful the death must have been. The three witnesses took less than two hours before they rested their case.

The judge called for a recess and we all stepped outside for air. Even though it was fall, the courtroom stifled. None of the windows was open.

"We need that girl," Robert said to me.

Mr. Weaver had tried to get Wade's friend to take the stand, but her family wouldn't allow it. They was too scared to get mixed up in it. Robert had visited with the family himself but couldn't persuade the daddy. It didn't help that the man didn't want nobody thinking his unmarried daughter was out at night messing around with a boy from the kingdom, even if his mama was the queen. But the girl was the only one who could vouch for Wade's whereabouts that night.

When we started up again, Mr. Weaver called Wade to the stand first and asked him flat outright if he let the bulls loose. Wade answered forcefully. "No, I did not." Then he asked him, "Did you kill that man?" Wade shook his head, adding, "I don't even hunt, Mr. Weaver. It ain't my way to kill none of God's creatures, whether accidental or on purpose."

The small crowd in the courtroom murmured at that, and I couldn't tell if they was impressed or found his unsolicited declaration unruly.

"Were you in Saluda that night, Mr. Montgomery?"

"Yes, sir."

"Why were you there?"

"I was there to see a friend. But she don't live nowhere near this farmer."

"Is it possible someone saw you walking home and thought you was coming from Mr. Roy's house?"

"I reckon they could have seen me. I wasn't trying to hide or nothing."

"That's all my questions, Your Honor."

Next the prosecutor was called up for cross-examination. "Who was this friend you were seeing that night?"

Wade's eyes jumped over to me and then back at the lawyer. "A young lady, sir."

"A lady! Okay." The lawyer turned to the jury and there was a titter of laughter among them. "And what might be this young lady's name?"

"Objection, Your Honor," said Mr. Weaver. "Clearly the defendant's young friend is not on the witness list, so there's no need to confirm her identity."

"Overruled. The whereabouts of your client that night are

crucial to this case, Mr. Weaver. You know that. Providing a name may lend credibility to his story."

Weaver sat down.

"Please answer the question, Mr. Montgomery."

I knew Wade didn't want to mention the girl's name because he wanted to protect her reputation. But I'd already told him that if he had to choose between his life and her name, he needed to choose his life. I leaned forward. *Say the name, Wade.*

"I-I would rather not say, sir."

The courtroom erupted.

"Order!" the judge demanded.

"Was there really a girl? Or did you make this girl up?"

"Objection!"

"No further questions, Your Honor." The prosecutor sat down.

Mr. Weaver stood again. "Mr. Montgomery, can you please inform the court why you're reluctant to provide a name."

"Why I'm what?"

"Why you don't want to say the girl's name."

"She's a nice girl, and I don't want nobody to get the wrong impression. We was just talking that night. We wasn't doing nothing wrong. She don't deserve all this attention."

I couldn't sit still. With him not sharing the girl's name, the jury might assume Wade had been with a white girl. They never associated honor with colored girls, didn't even think it was possible. My poor son was hammering the nail in his coffin ten different ways.

After Wade walked back to his seat, the lawyer called for William to take the stand. Sunny led him up to the stand by the hand.

"Could you state your name for the record?"

"William Montgomery."

"Mr. Montgomery, what is your relationship with the defendant?"

"He's my nephew, but he's like a son to me. I raised him as my own."

Robert tensed beside me, and I put a hand on his arm. Mr. Weaver had decided to call up William rather than Robert, probably thinking his lack of sight might draw sympathy from the jury.

"How old is Wade?"

"He's fifteen, sir."

"And what kind of boy is he?"

"Oh, he's like most boys, I imagine. He likes to be with his friends, likes to ride horses and talk to girls."

"Have you ever known him to lie?"

"Objection!"

William didn't wait for the judge to answer before responding, "Never in my life."

That was Mr. Weaver's only question for William. When the judge asked the prosecutor if he had questions for William, he waved his hand and said, "No, Your Honor."

After William's testimony, the defense rested and the judge called for closing arguments. I watched every move the lawyers made.

The kingdom council stepped outside and drank water from canteens. We was mostly quiet, our faces long with worry.

"How long you think they take?" I asked Robert.

Robert shook his head. He had a grave look in his eyes that I couldn't stand. "Not long enough for us to walk back up the hill."

He was right. We was just starting to pull out the food we'd packed when the court clerk came out to tell us the jury had reached a verdict.

We filed back in the courtroom and ordered ourselves in the back row. Vernon had arrived, and he squeezed in beside Sunny. Wade glanced back at us. William turned his head so he could hear everything. I began to rock from side to side. The judge shuffled papers. I looked over at the jury, the white men who would decide my son's fate. None of them would make eye contact with me. It reminded me of the day they'd beaten my papa down in Cross Anchor. The same firm set of the lip.

In just one day of trial, the jury found my Wade guilty and the judge sentenced him to two years in prison. Other than my papa's death, it was the darkest day of my life.

THIRTY-SIX

W̲e lost our land and our son. And by that, I mean to say we lost everything.

Mr. Weaver wanted us out so he could rent the houses. On a cold Sunday evening in November 1894, the council of the Kingdom of the Happy Land met for the final time. The young people had already started making plans about where they would go, but us people who had been there from the early days took our time. We'd always wondered when this day would come. The hope that we'd be able to hold on to that land forever began to die, reminding us how dangerous it was to dream.

So even though the kingdomfolk wasn't too happy, the look on their faces was one of resignation. We sat as usual near the oak tree. Me and Robert had woke up that morning and put on our fancy clothes. We'd even draped William in the king's cape. It was as if we wanted to say to ourselves that we would always be a royal people, no matter what.

"The lawyer man say we can raise the money to buy it back," Robert offered. "He give us a price and it's fair."

"How long you think it'll take y'all to get it saved up?" asked Billy Casey, Jola's brother.

"He give us two years," said Robert. It didn't matter how long it would take us. What mattered was how long we had before the lawyer's offer expired. Everybody knew that.

"I reckon I'll be on to glory by then," joked Reverend Couch. But no one laughed with him.

"Do everybody got somewhere to go?" asked William.

Jola answered. "Everybody except that young family from Tennessee. They ain't got family around here. We working on finding them a place."

"When they take the land, they might tear down the houses. If we buy it back, we got to start over," said Billy.

Robert shook his head. "No, the man say he plan to keep the houses and rent them out. But he say he sell it all back to us when we ready." He kept repeating this part of the deal, as if saying it over and over again would make it happen.

"Maybe he rent the houses to us?"

"He want to rent them to white families," I said.

Everybody sat with that for a minute. White families could pay more in rent than we could. The thought of our beloved kingdom handed right over like that wasn't easy to swallow.

"It's all my fault," I said.

"No, Lu, don't say that."

"I never should've agreed to pay with the land."

"We agreed. Not just you. And we ain't have a choice." Robert rubbed my back.

"What's done is done," William said. "We ain't got but forty or so people living on this mountain. Maybe it's time."

"You only need one person to hold the land," I said. "Just one that want to live here."

Somebody passed around a gourd of corn whiskey. We took turns drinking from it, even the women.

That night, we went to bed filled with memories of waking to birdsong, picking purple long-stemmed flowers, eating serviceberries and licking the stain from our teeth, hovering over sickbeds only to grieve with the families of the departed. Resting beside the creek on that mountain, we had found God's grace, the cool trickle of water like a baptism as we skated a toe across its surface. Up here, where it was so quiet you could hear a squirrel chew, we had worshipped and healed and cried and held forth in prayer and gratitude. That night, we all slept restless, every last one of us, tossing with the same dreams. This place wasn't just our home, it was our refuge.

Before we could leave, before we walked down that hill and passed through the gate for what might be the final time, there was some things we needed to do. Like finger the grooves in the walls of our cabins where we'd marked the growth of our children, slide a foot across a well-worn floor to recall its dusty feel, slice a piece of bark from the old oak, flatten a hand against the dirt that had fed us, drape ourselves in the speckled light that drizzled through the trees, visit the place where our people was buried. Pay respects in that sacred place where all the kingdom-folk who had passed over lay in eternal rest.

All this just to capture our memories, doing as we'd always done, putting them away, capping them lest they leak and destroy all the happiness we'd captured.

In that year of our Lord, 1894, nearly thirty years into freedom, hundreds of years after our people first landed on these shores, we lifted our arms to the sky. The kingdom had been more than grass, trees, and dirt—this land had the power, wonder-working healing power, to save us. It was God's promise to the poor in spirit, our kingdom of heaven, our treasure.

One by one, we packed up and left the mountain. It was fall and we picked everything we could from the ground that we could take with us, divided our stores of food. I said my goodbyes to the little cemetery, lay a flower on Papa's stone.

My one final hope, the only dream I allowed myself, was that right around the time Wade finished working in the camp we would be back in our house and I could welcome him home to his own bedroom upstairs in the palace. For two years, I would do nothing but work as I planned my son's homecoming. For two years, I would focus on getting everything back we had lost.

Morning, noon, and night.

Two years of scrimping and saving to buy back our land, two years of working hard as I had in slavery times, and I would have to sit down and tearfully have a serious talk with my god.

THIRTY-SEVEN

Nikki

The next morning, we dress for court. Mother Rita wears one of her church dresses and perches a hat on top of her thinning hair. Shawnie wears burgundy slacks and a silk blouse she once borrowed from me and never returned. Mama has painted her lips a flattering pink that matches her suit. I wear a dress unsuitable for the humidity.

We pile into Mother Rita's minivan. Someone has vacuumed up all the flower debris, and I briefly wonder if Bryan did the favor. A little over half an hour later, we park outside the Henderson County Courthouse, which is just a few blocks from Bryan's library. I look around for his car. He said he would meet us here, but I don't see him.

"What kind of lawyer is this?" Mama asks.

"I got the same question," Mother Rita chimes in. "She says she's a Casey."

"Tax and estate law," I answer. Though Mama sounds skeptical about the meeting, she was the first one of us to wake up this morning and put on coffee. After the previous night's drama, it has been a relief to see the two of them get along this morning, a chorus of unified voices on everything from what we would have for breakfast—cut-up fruit and toast—to where everyone would sit in the car—me and Shawnie in the front so the two older ladies could be chauffeured.

R.J. doesn't leave us waiting long, which is a gift because it feels as if the four of us are teetering on the edge of a cliff, our amicable truce ready to topple with one stray word. We meet R.J. in the lobby and she ushers us to a conference room she has reserved.

I watch Mother Rita, who appears too afraid to hope for good news. Mama is more unreadable, though I know she suspects this may be a ruse to charge us exorbitant legal fees. When I told her R.J. hasn't asked for a retaining fee, that only exaggerated her suspicion. *Today will be the money grab*, she is probably thinking.

Shawnie is pensive. Though I'm a little worried about her, I'm grateful she is here to be part of this experience, to learn about her family's history, no matter how it turns out.

R.J. sweeps into the room in her usual grand style, wearing a purple suit, her big hair immaculately teased. Typical D.C. lawyers are boring compared to R.J. She gives a lie to the notion of lawyers as staid and conservative. I think it's even more intriguing that she appears before a judge in all her glorious, unapologetic self.

"R.J., this is my grandmother Rita Lovejoy and my mother, Lorelle. My daughter, Shawnie."

"Oh, you're the one that just graduated high school. Where do you plan to go to college?"

Shawnie glances over at me. R.J. probably thinks she just graduated in June. She doesn't realize she has been out of high school for over a year.

"I plan to take some courses at UDC."

"Alright, then. I love D.C. In another life, I think I was born and raised there. Lucky you." I can definitely picture R.J. in my town shaking things up.

"Yes, ma'am," Shawnie says. Her bottom lip quivers a bit, and I can see that the question about college upsets her no matter who is asking it. It's the conversation at the bottom of much of our discord over the past year. I have been pushing her to either take classes or apply for a government job.

"My my my. Four generations," R.J. begins. "When Nikki texted me to tell me you'd all be here, I was so excited. And Mrs. Lovejoy, I am so happy to finally get a chance to meet you. Did she tell you I'm a Casey?"

"She did. Doris Casey's granddaughter?"

"Yes, ma'am. I grew up hearing about the kingdom. So for me, this is personal. That's why I told Nikki I wouldn't charge y'all one penny."

I glance quickly at Mama, but her face is blank, as if she isn't listening, though I know she is.

"Our hearing has been pushed back thirty minutes, so we have a little time to chat. Today we are strictly responding to the eviction notice and nothing else. Mrs. Lovejoy, it is my understanding you and your family have lived on the land for nearly a hundred fifty years, ever since the days of the kingdom."

"I was born on that property, as were the women before me."

"But you lost the land due to an heirs' property action a little over twenty years ago."

"Now, I may not have a legal claim to that property in your world, Mrs. Parker, but I got my rights."

R.J. offers Mother Rita an understanding smile. She is finally meeting Rita Lovejoy in the flesh and witnessing firsthand the stubbornness I've been managing.

"You tell that judge that I am a direct descendant of the Kingdom of the Happy Land and Queen Luella Montgomery."

When Mother Rita says this, Mama interrupts. "Mrs. Parker, are you planning to ask the judge to allow Mama to stay there temporarily given her . . . extenuating circumstances?"

"Exactly right. I expect their counsel to object to the request, so I'm hoping to garner even more sympathy given Mrs. Lovejoy's longtime familial connection to the land. I see no reason the Thomas brothers can't hold off on the sale a little while longer. They've waited all this time."

"There's no need to talk about the kingdom, is there? I mean, we know our family lived there, established a community, and bought acreage. That's enough," Mama says.

Mama is so transparent in her disbelief. No wonder Mother Rita got fed up with her. I'm not sure when I became a believer, but I am. All Mama has to do is open her mind to the same kind of imagination Luella had. It must have taken such belief in the magic of possibility for those kingdomfolk to call themselves royals. Somewhere along the way, our family had lost that wonder. Maybe that's what's wrong with Shawnie.

Oh, Mama, I want to say.

"If you'd been around here long enough, you'd know the locals all heard of the kingdom, Lorelle. She should mention it," says Mother Rita.

"That judge is going to think you're crazy," Mama snaps back. "And the lawyers will use that to argue that's why they're having trouble evicting you, all because of some batshit story—"

"Watch your mouth, Lorelle Lovejoy."

"It's Lorelle Berry. I haven't been a Lovejoy in years."

"No, you haven't," Mother Rita says quietly.

No one in the room speaks or moves for a full minute. R.J. is looking sheepishly at the paper in front of her, perhaps wondering if she should excuse herself. I'm sure she has witnessed bickering families before. The poison between Mama and Mother Rita has festered so long that it taints the air in the room. I can taste it.

"So just to recap," R.J. starts up again carefully, "my plan is to ask the judge to grant you some leniency given your family history with the land. If he gives us more time, Nikki can get to work on drawing up a contract offer to purchase. We'll keep it sweet and simple. How does that sound?"

"It sounds like a terrible idea. I don't understand why my granddaughter has to use her hard-earned money to buy land that already rightfully belongs to us."

I don't say anything. I haven't asked Mama about the possibility of taking out a line of credit on her house. She knows I don't have the money, so she looks over at me curiously.

R.J. glances at me. "Mrs. Lovejoy, I've told your granddaughter this, but I have to reiterate it now. I'd be doing you a disservice if I weren't completely straight up with you. You do not have a lawful claim to the land at this point other than by purchasing it back. I'm so sorry."

Mother Rita breathes in through her nose. "The nerve of those men. Serving me notice to vacate at my age."

No one says anything. Shawnie blinks furiously. I can tell she's about to cry. Even Mama is looking down at her lap. Mother Rita's voice is thick with indignation.

309

"The only other option here is to resolve this through arbitration. I'm not sure it would work, though. Nikki tried to talk to Albert Thomas, but he says his brother is unwilling to negotiate."

Mother Rita rises abruptly and leaves the room. We sit in the funk of her outrage. This has all got to be so upsetting. I'm about to go after her when Mama says, "Nikki, how on earth are you planning to make an offer on this property?"

R.J. finally excuses herself. "I'll go see after Mrs. Lovejoy."

I smile thinly as we wait for her to leave.

"So?"

"I was thinking you could take out a second mortgage on the house." I sound like a child, telling my mother how to spend her money.

"Nikki, I already mortgaged the property years ago. I don't have the equity anymore."

"Wait, what?" She did this without telling me? I thought Mama and I shared everything. My first thought is: I can't believe Mama took out a second mortgage without consulting me and my trusted list of lenders. My second thought is: We don't have the money to buy the land. I've failed Mother Rita and generations of my family. I'm still reeling with this news and what it means when R.J. sticks her head in the door. "I think we should make our way to the courtroom. Our hearing should be next on the docket. Y'all ready?"

It's time to go face the Thomas brothers. And no, I am not ready.

THIRTY-EIGHT

Luella

After leaving the kingdom, I moved with Robert and William to Sunny and Vernon's new home. Faced with the prospect of the kingdom disbanding, Vernon rented five acres of land in Flat Rock with a main house and a one-room cabin. Me and Robert moved into the cabin. William lived in the main house with Sunny and Vernon, and he began to do for the young couple what he had once done for our home in the kingdom and for the men in the mining camp. Each morning, he swept and cleaned up for Sunny, who helped her husband in the field.

Though our days was filled with anguish over our son's absence, me and Robert delighted in getting to know each other again. At night he held me in his arms, the lovemaking more tender and generous than it had ever been. I was back with the man I'd loved more than life. Once again Robert was my chosen one.

On a square of land near our cabin I hoed rows for flowers, and that first spring, my roses blossomed. I planted a row of sunflowers right outside my window, and sometimes, Robert would cut a few and put them in a glass on the table. They was our favorites, reminders of our fields of sun on the mountain.

I sold flowers around town, and Robert began to repair shoes, using the skills he'd learned years before from the shoemaker. In the evening after he got home, we would sit in the backyard and look out over the flowers while swatting flies bold enough to land right on our noses. It wasn't the mountain—Flat Rock was on a plateau—but it was pretty land and we found visions of joy in it. We was still outdoors people, living by the weather vane.

Word came down the hill that families was living up there in our houses and the gate was wide open. Now anybody with two feet could walk right up in there. We heard the lawyer had even put a little store up on the mountain so the tenants didn't have to go all the way to town. I had to admit it was a good idea, but it was enough to put a hurting on my heart.

What kept us going was the knowledge that we was putting our money away. And watching the date of Wade's return kept our eyes lifted to the sky. As much as we loved Vernon and Sunny's place, me and Robert wanted to leave them be so they could focus on growing their family. Plus, the little cabin was small, and though it was fine for the time being, we missed our palace in the kingdom. We heard the new owners had run electric wires up the mountain, and Robert promised me that if they hadn't done it already, when we returned he would put electric lightbulbs in our house just like what Vernon and Sunny had in theirs. I imagined all that I could do at night with a lightbulb.

The closer we got to Wade's release date, the more I began to feel something was wrong. I told Robert I was afraid they might not let him go. We hadn't been able to visit him because Wade worked on a farm called Caledonia that was hundreds of miles away. We couldn't work and save and visit him, too. We had heard from a man who had heard from a man who had just come back that the work wasn't no different from plantation labor, and the thought sickened me. I knew about slavery times, but my child had been born free and he didn't know nothing about the lash. The man told us he had met men there who would work at the camp for the rest of their natural-born days. I was just thankful my boy had an end date.

Robert and William started spending time together, going for walks after Robert come back to the house in the evening and sitting on the porch of the house talking while William spat chewing tobacco into the dirt. The brothers was back together again, healing in their own way.

As the date of Wade's release drew nearer, we decided we would celebrate. Some of the women Sunny had grown up with in the kingdom helped us plan for the feast. We fattened up a hog and a few chickens that winter, lay aside flour for bread.

One morning, I stepped out of my little house and looked up at the sky, just to make sure it was still blue. I'd learned that as long as the sky kept its promise, there was still life to be lived. I wiped my damp forehead and then looked up, startled to see Sunny running up the hill.

"Ma! Pa!" she yelled out.

I braced myself for news. That kind of hollering could only mean she had something to tell us. And it didn't look like news of a grandchild fast as she was running.

"I got a letter! It's from Wade!"

I wiped my palms down the front of my apron. "A letter?" I yelled at her as Robert came up behind me and put a palm against my back.

313

Sunny stopped and sank to her knees in the grass. She ripped open the envelope and read it silently. I was too afraid to ask what it said. If Wade's name was on the envelope, he couldn't be dead. So maybe he was writing to tell us he wasn't coming home after all. I remembered the news that William had been hurt in the mines. Was my son hurt?

Sunny grinned.

"He on his way home, Ma. He say he reckon the letter get here before he will, but he want you to know that he is coming home early."

Tears ran down my face. I didn't know what else to do other than just let them flow. My boy was coming home early? I couldn't even form my lips to ask *when*. I was still trying to understand.

All I could say was, "The hog ain't ready yet."

THIRTY-NINE

R obert took Delight to Etowah to meet Wade and bring him to our place in Flat Rock. Days had passed since Robert left, and I waited at the door impatiently. I still couldn't believe this was happening. When the two of them finally started up the foot-path to the house, Sunny started yelling. "They here! They here!"

I ran up to the house where Sunny, Vernon, and William was already lined up on the porch. Robert tied the mule to the post and walked ahead, as if too excited to wait for Wade, who was walking like one leg was shorter than the other. I wiped my forehead with the sleeve of my dress. I had promised myself I wouldn't cry.

But when Wade walked up to me and I put my arms around his waist, feeling the muscle beneath his shirt, the beard on his chin, a lump rose in my chest.

"Hey, Ma," he said.

I touched his eyebrow. "Is it really you? You so tall now." Taller than his daddies.

The old Wade would've teased me back, would've called me

short. But this new man standing in front of me barely smiled. He just whispered, "I missed you, Ma."

And it was him crying, not me, as I brought his head down to my shoulder. "You home now, son. You with your family now."

Sunny hugged both of us. "Your letters was too short! Had us worried half to death," she said.

Finally, he revealed a glimpse of his old self. "And how was I supposed to read your handwriting, girl? Look like a chicken wrote it."

"Boy, you sure is a Montgomery!" William said, touching the top of Wade's head. No doubt about it, the boy had grown what looked like half a foot in two years.

I wouldn't let Wade out of my sight over the next few days. And he seemed to want to stay near me, too. When he walked by, I pulled him to me and put a hand to his cheek. Unlike when he was younger, he didn't pull away, as if he needed the touching much as I did.

"They treat you alright?" I asked him once.

"Yes, Ma," he said, though I knew he was sparing me the worst.

"They fed you?"

"They fed us alright. It didn't taste like nothing, not like king-dom food."

"You make a friend or two?"

"I ain't never going to forget them men, Ma."

"I prayed for you," I said to him once when he was helping me clear the weeds in my garden. Robert and William had both forced him to sit for a while before finding work. Their son had done nothing but work for the last two years, and though he had filled out as a man, the outline of muscles stretching his shirtsleeves tight, his two daddies wanted him to do nothing for a change. Work was always just around the corner for a young man like him, but the pleasure of rest was something we'd learned in the kingdom.

Once Wade tired of sitting around, he offered to help me in my garden. I didn't ask him what kind of work he'd done on the farm, but I didn't have to. I'd grown up on a plantation and knew its secrets.

Sunny said Wade woke early every morning, even earlier than Vernon, who was usually in the fields by sunrise. When Sunny fed him, he cleaned his plate and asked for more. At night, she could hear him moaning as he slept, and she'd caught William sitting in the chair next to his bed. Just sitting there beside him in the dark. Sunny shared all this with me when I asked her how Wade was doing up in the main house, which I asked every single day.

I noticed something new in my son, my mother's eyes as alert as ever. There was a scar beneath his left eye, and a patch in his hair that had not grown back. When he wasn't shoving them in his pockets, his hands shook. I watched him now, his hands deep in the dirt of my garden patch.

"Pass me that rake."

"Ma, can I ask you a question?"

It was nearing the end of the season, and most of my flowers was finished. Everything left was something fit for the table. Turnips, cabbage, pole beans, squash. "Course, son."

"What happened to the kingdom? Ain't nobody told me why we left."

I pulled the rake lightly over the dirt. Next year, I would see about planting some of them dahlias Jola was growing over at her place.

"I suppose wasn't nobody left but the council?"

I planted the rake in the ground. The middle of the day was

upon us, and it had warmed up enough to be pleasant. "We paid for the lawyer with the land."

"My lawyer?"

"Yes."

He said nothing, but I could sense his sadness. We'd planned to have the kingdom back before Wade returned. No one had been prepared for him to come home six months early.

"It ain't so bad. When we pay him, we'll get the land back. We almost there with the money. I been keeping a careful eye on the book. Pretty soon, we'll be back in the palace."

"I heard it's white folk living up there now."

"The man that's holding it just renting them out for now. We get it back soon."

"Ma."

"It's alright, son."

My voice sounded strong, but Wade's questions got me to thinking. The council hadn't met for a few months, but we was due to meet that next month, and if all went according to our plan, we could be back in the kingdom by Christmas.

That night, I told Robert we needed to go see the lawyer, who was still in the same office on Main Street. We needed to let him know we was ready to draw up the papers to pay him and get our land back.

Robert sat on the bed. The light was waning. I couldn't wait for them electric lightbulbs. I wondered if the people living in my house had already put some lightbulbs in my bedroom.

"We need to wait for the council meeting, talk to Billy, make sure we all in agreement."

"Last time it took Mr. Weaver weeks to draw up them papers. I want to be back in my house by Christmas."

"It ain't nothing but October now. We meet in a few weeks. Then we go see him."

But I wouldn't settle. Day after day, I worried Robert about it.

How in the world is Sunny going to get pregnant with Wade and William wandering around the house all day?

What if Mr. Weaver going to visit family for the holidays and ain't got time to write the papers before the new year?

Ooh, this cabin small. Don't you miss having stairs?

I wonder if them people cut down some of our trees. Remember old Bertha, the poplar behind our house that turned so orange every fall it would blind you?

Remember when Delight ate them berries out back and her stomach got all messed up?

I was thinking Wade could take one of the houses. Maybe find himself a wife.

Finally, Robert agreed that we would go visit with the lawyer before the council meeting.

FORTY

Nikki

The morning after the hearing, early as the birds rise, I join Mama and Mother Rita in the gardens while Shawnie sleeps in. Zinnias are still blooming, and though they'll all be gone by the first frost, their little buds hold the promise of summer's end. Mother Rita missed the flower market the day before because of the hearing, but she will deliver to a few local churches this weekend.

We set a stool on the row for Mother Rita to sit while she works. I spread out a pallet of tools beside her, and when she is ready to move down the row, I move her stool and tools and reposition her. Mama keeps her distance, but from what I can tell, she has a practiced hand with the flowers. In fact, it's clear she knows how to do all the things Mother Rita can do. Why did I never know this?

At the end of the row, Mama waits for me. She goes into the toolshed and comes back with a blanket. She spreads it on the ground and sits on it. I sit beside her, near its edge. Mother Rita keeps working, and we watch her lazily, speaking low enough that we are just out of earshot.

"I can't believe you took out a second mortgage," I say.

"I wish I could buy it for her, Nikki. Even if we bought it, what would we do with it? It's too late now."

"Too late for us to hold the land our family worked so hard to protect? It only takes one person."

"And who would that be? You?"

"You still don't believe in the kingdom," I say.

"Does it matter what I believe?"

"I think it does, Mama."

My grandmother rises from the stool and stretches her arms. Then she moves the stool, sits again, and continues working. Her hair is wrapped in a white cotton cloth and her brown face beams against the bright fabric.

I look at my mama. She is so much like Mother Rita—the determination, the unembellished truth. I imagine Luella might have been the same. Or maybe she was pliant like me, finding herself a leader when she least expected it. Sitting here beside the garden on this August day, I feel the spirit of Luella alongside us.

"Mama, you know what was the first thing I realized after I truly believed my great-great-great-grandmother was a queen?"

She turns to me and tilts her head.

"I realized that maybe I would've done different if I'd known I was descended from royalty. Maybe I would've gone to college or dreamed bigger. Maybe I would've understood that the possibilities for my future were limitless."

"Nikki, your daddy and I never denied you anything. You could've done anything you wanted—"

"Mama, you can't do it if you can't imagine it!"

My voice carries but Mother Rita doesn't look over at us. She continues deadheading, dropping flowers into the bucket beside her.

"I always thought our family stopped dreaming after Daddy died. But now I know we stopped long before that."

Mama looks off into the woods.

"Those kingdom people walked up that mountain, fleeing violence, daring to make their own community. They grew their own food, bartered, traded, pooled their resources, and made a life. They bought a little over two hundred acres and then fought like hell to hold on to it. Now we've lost it. All because we didn't believe."

"Nikki—"

"What are y'all over there chattering on about?" Mother Rita calls out as she makes her way to us. She places her stool next to the blanket and straightens out her legs. We all sit in silence for a few minutes. My grandmother is taking all of this remarkably well. After the judge ruled that she had already been given adequate notice to vacate and would only be allowed seventy-five days to move out of her house, Mother Rita hadn't shed a single tear. It was as if she just began to focus on the next life.

But the ruling is weighing on all of us. It's a miracle we are even out here together this morning. It's time for us to start making arrangements, and we all know it.

"I'll stay here and help you get packed up, Mother Rita. Maddie Mae is fixing up her extra bedroom. She says you can stay with her until . . ."

"Until I'm dead. Just say it." Mother Rita takes off her gloves. "We all headed that way one day. Now, I've written down my wishes for when I'm gone. Check my bedside table drawer for my instructions. I got some life insurance. It's not a lot, but Shawnie's my beneficiary. Hopefully, it will motivate her to do something useful with her life."

"Mother Rita, we got to ask if they'll let us fence in the cem-

etery if you still want to be buried there next to Granddaddy—"
I interrupt.

She issues one of those sharp "tshh" sounds and presses a finger to her lips. "It's in my notes, but I may as well tell it now. Make sure I'm wearing my pretty orange dress. That's right, orange. And I want a white casket. If I pass in the dead of winter, it won't be a whole lot to choose from, but you can use greenery. Just don't use that fake mess. If I sense one fake flower anywhere near me, I'm rising back up and snatching somebody."

Mother Rita continues with her instructions, and soon her voice floats into a litany of dos and don'ts, until it is about more than a funeral and death plans and how to bury a matriarch. Lessons I've missed not growing up here and lessons that bear repeating for my mother, who lost her connection to this place long ago, and lessons for Shawnie, who will one day hear them from her mother and grandmother, long after Mother Rita rests beside her husband and ancestors.

"And I got burial insurance. Herbert paid it off before he passed." She pauses, as if that is all she can remember at the moment.

"I'm really sorry for not being there for you when you needed me." Mama's voice shakes, and I want to put an arm around her. But I've been shushed. Foolishly, as if I'm still a child, I don't want to make any sudden moves out of fear they'll send me in the house. These are the moments I've missed in my life, the sacredness of being in the presence of the elder matriarchs, and I am moved by the humility of it.

"You had every right to refuse, Lorelle. I shouldn't have said those ugly things to you. I should've called you back and apologized."

Mama puts her head in her hands.

Mother Rita goes on. "I just wanted you to show up for me,

prove you loved me. That wasn't right, I know that now. No daughter should have to hold up her mother's feelings."

"Mama—" she gasps. It is the first time I have heard my mama refer to Mother Rita that way, and I am shocked. We all hold still, even the wind, even the earth.

"And one more thing," Mother Rita is saying. "It's time for Veronica to know the truth."

My eyelid twitches. I put a finger to it to still the movement, though I know I look weird, as if I'm stopping a tear.

"You tell it," says Mama.

"You're the one kept it from her, Lorelle."

I am too frightened to move, let alone speak. What will be the lesson now? *This is how you open up a box of secrets for a daughter and free her. This is how you relieve yourself of the burden of carrying that secret. This is how you end a generation of mistakes.*

"Nikki," Mama begins. She pauses for a moment, gathering herself. "After your daddy died, Mother Rita called and asked me to help with the property taxes. I had some life insurance money and she knew it. But I refused. I didn't believe in the old kingdom story, and I thought she should give up the house and move closer to us. The Thomas family were the rightful owners of the land by that time, but your grandmother wouldn't budge. She had been paying the property taxes as if it was still her land."

I frown at Mama.

"Don't look at me like that. I figured I'd eventually pay it if she pushed back hard enough. I thought if I stalled, she might give up and come live with me in D.C. I didn't realize she was already months late with the payment when she reached out to me. In the meantime, the county tracked down and notified the Thomas brothers about the late payment. We ran out of time."

"And that's how they discovered they owned the land," I fill in. "Because she didn't pay the taxes on time. They never even knew they'd inherited it from their daddy twelve years before when he died."

"You got it," says Mother Rita.

"I felt terrible about the whole thing, but there was nothing I could do. Within weeks, they sent out a surveyor."

"If she'd just paid when I asked her, we wouldn't even be in this mess."

"Mother Rita, they would've eventually found out," Mama says.

"Found out what? That their daddy stole this land right out from under us?"

"The land was already gone. You lost this land twenty years ago."

"And you found that unforgivable, Mother Rita?" I look at my grandmother. "Because she refused to pay?"

"Tell her everything, Lorelle." Mother Rita looks over at her daughter. "Tell her what you said to me when you left here at eighteen years old. Tell her how you disrespected this land and everything it stood for. Tell her how many times over the years you called me foolish for believing in fairy tales. Tell her."

Mama doesn't say anything, but her face crumples. I know enough now to understand how long their discord has been festering. This deep hurt between them has everything to do with their love for each other, but it also has everything to do with a long-ago queen who defied belief. The two women had literally erected a mountain between them, a mountain that had once nourished and sustained our people.

FORTY-ONE

Luella

On a Saturday morning in late October, we hitched the mule to the cart and rode to town. Saturday was a day that a lot of people did their shopping and took care of business, so Main Street was filled with folk hurrying off to one place or another. The center of town had changed so much in recent years. We even had an opera house, though I had never seen the inside of it. Everybody was talking about the new bank, a two-story brick building at the corner of Main Street and Fourth Avenue. I hadn't been inside because coloreds wasn't allowed. As we rode through town, I knew that all these changes was due to the railroad. It had changed everything.

We hitched Delight right outside of Mr. Weaver's office. The same woman sat at the desk, her hair still stretched back behind her ears.

"Mr. Weaver is in a meeting right now. Y'all want to come back this afternoon?"

"No, ma'am, we'll wait." I sat in the chair. This time, Robert sat down beside me.

I didn't know why she asked us to come back that afternoon, because it wasn't long before Mr. Weaver exited his office with another man who was replacing his hat. They exchanged pleasantries, and when Mr. Weaver saw us it was as if a cloud passed over his eyes.

"Mr. and Mrs. Montgomery, please come in."

We entered his office. There was a new desk, and the blinds that had been pulled before was now open, allowing for more sunlight.

"How may I help you today?"

"Well," Robert began, "we approaching the two-year mark on our land and we wanted to let you know we meeting with our council next month and . . ."

"Your land?"

Robert appeared flustered. "Your land, Mr. Weaver. It's your land, for sure, but we plan to pay you just like we agreed. We figure we come on down here so you can get the paperwork together cause my wife here is saying she want to be back on the land by Christmas."

I nodded. "My boy is home. Maybe you heard?"

"Yes, I heard. Congratulations."

"Thank you. We sure got you to thank for making sure he didn't die in that jail, but thank God he came home a little early. We got you to thank for that, too, I reckon."

"That's nice to hear, Mrs. Montgomery. I try to do my best." He turned to stare out the window and was silent for a few minutes.

Robert glanced at me and back at the lawyer. "Mr. Weaver, we know you got families living there, so if you need some time to clear them . . ."

I coughed. We'd just said we wanted to be back by Christmas, and here was Robert offering the man more time.

327

"You know, Mr. Montgomery, it ain't easy being a small-town lawyer. We don't have a lot of trials here, and I don't make a lot of money doing papers for people. I could make a whole lot more money if I moved to the city, I reckon."

Me and Robert remained quiet. We didn't know nothing about what he was talking.

"My grandson Charlie married now. I give him and his wife a new house for their wedding."

"That's a mighty fine thing to do for them," Robert said. I was wondering if the new house was on our property, and from the tone of his voice, I knew Robert was wondering the same.

"He about the same age as your Wade, if I remember correctly. But he got a nice wife who say she want to have ten babies. She already carrying! Ain't that something. I am going to be a great-grandfather come springtime."

"Congratulations, sir."

My eyes clouded. He couldn't be saying what I thought he was saying. He'd promised.

"So when my boy tell me he is going need a house and some property, you know what I done? I looked around town to see what I could buy. Something right here in Hendersonville where my wife could see the new baby anytime she want."

"Here in Hendersonville?" I whispered. The kingdom wasn't in Hendersonville. What was he saying?

"We built him a house with twelve rooms. I never seen something so grand."

I could hear Robert swallowing. So the lawyer hadn't moved his son into our palace. I tried to decipher his words.

"What I'm saying is I got family to take care of. Surely you understand that."

My voice sounded small in my ears. "How much, Mr. Weaver?"

All this time Robert had been gazing out the window. Now he turned back to face us, his chair scraping the floor. The lawyer wrote a number on a piece of paper and handed it to Robert.

"Course I'll give you more time to come up with the money. But it's only fair, don't you think? Your boy is home now. Without me, he might be swinging from a tree. I made sure nobody touched him, and he only spent eighteen months for a murder. I'd say that's pretty good."

Robert grabbed my hand and squeezed it so hard that it hurt. I knew it was a warning, because I couldn't see straight. My eyes was blurring, but I had to catch myself. I could feel Robert willing his strength into me, urging me to calm.

I didn't even have to look at the number to know it was impossible.

On the way back to Vernon and Sunny's house, neither Robert nor I could bear to speak, let alone look at one another. Mr. Weaver knew the judges and everybody else who was the law in Henderson County. We was powerless to stop him.

When we arrived back at the palace, we stayed in the cart, just sitting there as the sun dipped out of the sky. As if aware we wasn't to be disturbed, the mule waited patiently. Finally, we roused at the sound of her emptying her bladder.

"We got to borrow the money," Robert said. "If we wait another two years, the price will change again."

"Borrow from who?" I said. "The bank will never loan it to us, and even if they did, I don't trust them."

"The Widow's son. We borrow the money from him and pay Weaver. Better to be in debt to Davis."

I breathed in and out, going over the idea in my mind. The

plan could work if the Widow's son loaned us the money. But we'd be paying him back a long time. Weaver had given us a price high enough for him to keep the land forever.

"What if the Widow's son don't loan it to us?" I asked. That man never did like us, and even though his mama had loved our liniment, bought my flowers, and called on us when she got sick, he didn't have the same regard for us. I calculated the price per acre, what Weaver was really asking in his inflated new number. The South Carolina land was a bunch of forest, but it was good timber and soil.

"We got enough money for fifty acres." I was thinking aloud. "Let's just buy back the kingdom settlement." What we really wanted was the houses, the stream, the graveyard holding our loved ones. Weaver might be satisfied with undeveloped land, especially since he was basically stealing it from us.

"And lose all that land we worked so hard for? We'd be losing over a hundred and fifty acres. No, Lu. We got to find another way."

I turned to look at Robert. He hadn't been around the kingdom since I became the leader. He wasn't used to seeing me take the reins. He didn't know how I ruled with the love and conviction taught to me by my papa. "Fifty acres is still more than what we came up here with," I told him. "Fifty acres is still enough to make a life. Fifty acres is fifty acres. If we get that portion back, we hold on to it and never let it go ever again, no matter what happens. Then we don't owe nobody. We still free."

I was going to be in my house by Christmas. So help me.

FORTY-TWO

Nikki

The gathering of the four of us had not been an easy visit, but we somehow got through it. Mama and Shawnie returned home, and I stayed behind to help Mother Rita pack up. I received an offer on the D.C. rowhouse that was just under listing price, and my clients accepted it. I wrote up the contract while still in Hendersonville, and Darius will handle the closing. Much to Mother Rita's delight, I'll be here taking care of her as long as she needs me.

I'm surprised at how good it feels to have more alone time with my grandmother. We work in the garden each day to finish the final harvesting and last few weeks of market vending before the land is turned over to the Thomas brothers. I'm proud of how quickly I'm learning. I've even bought new shoes. Mother Rita has taught me how to bake a fresh loaf of bread, and it's so tasty that I sell a few loaves at the market.

Each week, Stephen and Bryan help set up, and together we are managing to close out the season. A few days ago, Bryan gifted me a pair of binoculars. I wear them around my neck all the time, even when I'm gardening, hoping to catch a few bird sightings be-fore the fall migration picks up. When I think of Bryan, I find myself smiling.

I'm trying to maintain Mother Rita's strength and spirits, so whenever she has the energy, we walk a little ways along the trail in the woods, me holding her arm and listening to her tell me ev-erything she remembers her mother, Lily, sharing about our fam-ily. I think the most shocking detail is that Luella was supposedly in love with both Montgomery brothers. It's salacious! And actu-ally, I have to admit, kind of modern and badass.

We keep busy to fight our sadness at losing the land. Mother Rita doesn't talk about it, but I can tell she is saying goodbye a little bit each day. Sometimes she just stops and stares, and I don't know what she's looking at. I wait for her to gather herself before we continue with whatever we are doing. At night, I tuck her in as if she is a child, refilling her water glass and returning to turn off the lamp once she has fallen asleep with a book on her chest.

One afternoon, my grandmother, looking a little more tired than usual, excuses herself to rest in her room. I decide to watch television in the sunroom.

My cell phone buzzes just as I'm settling down on the sofa.

"Nikki, it's R.J."

"Hey."

R.J. had been right about the judge—she was kind and sympathetic—but she still ordered Mother Rita to vacate. It was a cruel outcome for our family, but a fair one in the eyes of the law. We are grateful to R.J. for her help.

"I woke up the other morning thinking about the fact that Fred Thomas has been dead twenty years," R.J. says.

"Okay."

"In North Carolina law, there's something called adverse possession. If a person occupies a property for a certain length of time, in an open and notorious fashion, while improving upon the land and living on it as if it's their own, they can claim title. I mean, it's a little more complicated than that, but that's basically it."

"Adverse possession? I've heard of that, but mainly when it comes to a dispute over a fence that has encroached on the neighbor's property. I didn't know you could claim title of an entire property if you're a hostile occupant."

"Something like that. The law uses words like *hostile* and *notorious*, but really it all just means openly and without permission."

"And are you telling me the statutory period in North Carolina for claiming title through adverse possession is twenty years?"

"Exactly right. I think Mother Rita fits all the requirements. She has never left the land since Thomas passed away, which means she has been there for at least twenty years."

Surely this is a Hail Mary. "Could that actually work?" I ask her.

"Yes, I think it could work."

I stop breathing for a moment. "Oh my goodness, R.J. Why didn't we think of this before?"

"I'm sorry, but I've never done this kind of claim. It's not too late, though."

"That judge was reasonable, but she was pretty strict in her interpretation of the law."

"That's the thing. This is legal, just like forced partition sales. We'd basically be doing the same thing Fred Thomas did—that is, using the law to force a transfer of the deed—but it would be to right the wrong he did to your family."

I glance toward the hallway and lower my voice. "I don't want to get Mother Rita's hopes up."

"I think she could use a little hope, don't you?"

"Yes, she really could."

After we hang up, every cell in my body is telling me that R.J. is onto something. It just might work. My first thought is to wonder how long it will take. I should've asked R.J. that question. I don't think Mother Rita has a lot of time left, and I'd want her to be here to see how it turns out. I'm hoping she will live until Christmas, just as she wishes.

"Why are you sitting in here looking like you just saw a ghost?" Mother Rita's voice is weaker but she still manages to project strength when she wants to.

"Oh, you're awake. You might as well sit down. I've got something to tell you that you are not going to believe."

Mother Rita smiles at me a little, as if she can already guess that I'm about to tell her the news she has been waiting for.

FORTY-THREE

The judge issues a temporary stay on the eviction until she can hear our new motion. It takes two months before we're able to get in front of her again. When the day of the hearing arrives, Mother Rita says she is too tired to attend, so I ask Bryan to take the day off and go with me. When he picks me up, he's dressed in a navy suit. He's always neat, but today he looks strikingly handsome.

"If this works, I hope she lives to see it," he says.

Bryan and I have so many things in common, and loving Mother Rita is just one of them. In fact, sitting in the car next to him, savoring the excitement of the day together, makes me realize something has snuck up on me. I like this man.

He takes my hand, casually, as if it is the most natural thing in the world, as if he's feeling the same way I am. I try not to look down at our interlocked fingers.

"What will you do with the land if you get to keep it?" he asks softly.

"That's a big if."

"Nikki, would you—"

"I can't move here, Bryan. My whole life is in D.C."

He laughs. "I wasn't going to say that, but now that you mention it."

Outside the window, the hills gently nest into each other. This North Carolina countryside opens me up in ways I can't explain. No wonder Luella loved two men. She looked out into this never-ending sky and all she wanted to do was love and be loved.

"You've said yourself that Shawnie is an adult now and it's time for her to make her own decisions." He's making a hard case now, but I'm listening. "You've admitted you're tired of real estate. I think you could do something with this land."

"We don't have the title yet. We could be kicked out of the house before the court even resolves it."

"But just imagine for a moment that y'all do get it." He glances over at me. "Just imagine."

I'm silent as I think of what I could do. The farmer's market is wonderful, but maybe I could do something bigger, like open my own business. My brain can't help but get stuck in the numbers of it. After all, I am an accountant's daughter. One thing I do know: I love being out there in the garden. It has become my happy place.

"I could open a nursery," I say, feeling a rush of inspiration. "A specialty place for flower lovers. I could even build a greenhouse."

"I'd help you. I'd be here every weekend, every day off, rain or shine."

The vision begins to form in my mind. Maybe even Miss Maddie could help. Her grandson, Stephen, loves being out there, too. What if I could pay him? I haven't seen a nursery anywhere near here, and even if there is, we'd be a family business.

"I could call it Kingdom Nursery?"

"Yes," he says and squeezes my fingers. "That would be a perfect name."

BRYAN DROPS ME back at the house that afternoon, leaving me to deliver the news without him. But I wasn't expecting company. Mother Rita and Maddie Mae are in the garden. I can hear their voices as soon as I step out the back door. I wonder if Mother Rita was really too tired to attend the hearing or if she was just nervous the judge would rule against us. I follow the sounds of the women, and over the fence I can see their heads moving down the rows. The two of them are giggling uncontrollably, sharing something that has them in stitches.

I unlatch the gate and enter the garden. Most of the flowers with blossoms have been cut, and there isn't much color left. It's early November and the wind is chilly. Normally, fall would have been vegetable planting season, but this year Mother Rita hasn't planted anything as she prepares to move out. I watch as she pulls her jacket around her and points at something on the ground. As I approach, I can see they are watching a rabbit who has stopped right in front of them. Mother Rita crouches down on her impossibly agile knees and holds out a piece of dry grass. The rabbit approaches and takes a nibble.

"Rita, that's probably the same rabbit that eats your black-eyed Susans," says Maddie Mae.

Mother Rita turns serious. "Doesn't make a bit of difference now, does it? They'll destroy this garden soon as they take possession."

I clear my throat and walk closer. Mother Rita stands and

337

turns. The two of them look so young out here, like schoolgirls. There is something about being in this garden that feels magical. Even without all the blossoms, it is still a special place where two elderly women become young again and rabbits appear suddenly at their feet. Behind us, the trees are a tapestry of yellow and brown, their rustling sounds like hands rubbing together in anticipation. When I look at Mother Rita now, the look of painful resignation, there is no question. She didn't go to court this morning because she couldn't bear it.

"The judge listened to everything R.J. had to say. It really was something to hear," I begin. "She told the story of the kingdom, presented the deed. She even told about how her own ancestor Jola Casey was a friend of our Queen Luella. Then she carefully walked through how each generation of the family has lived on the land and passed it down to the descendants. After Fred Thomas took it from us, she told how the Thomas family had neglected the land over the years. Even after the brothers knew they had inherited it, they didn't do anything with it."

"Look at God," Maddie Mae whispers.

"And when it came time, the judge didn't deliberate long before she issued her ruling." I pause. R.J. had called it complicated, but the claim feels simple to me. Mother Rita has lived here continuously all these years. It's her land. When I think about it, it's the very thing she has been saying to me all this time.

Mother Rita opens her mouth, then closes it. For once, she is not quick to speak.

I pass her an envelope. She takes it but doesn't open it. She just holds it in both hands, her eyes still on me. "That's a note from R.J. congratulating you. Mother Rita, the judge ruled that you are the rightful owner of four acres here that include your house, garden, the cemetery, and the entire road frontage. It's not everything, but it's something."

Mother Rita presses the envelope to her chest. I am nervous for a moment because I wonder if she is pleased. Darius had mentioned buying back the four acres that Mother Rita actually uses, so I'd suggested that number of acres to R.J. in our adverse possession motion and she'd agreed. It turned out to be the right idea, because the judge had not taken long to make her decision.

"Mother Rita? Are you happy with this outcome?"

She presses the unopened envelope back in my hand and wraps me in a hug, whispering in my ear. "The question is . . . are you happy, Nikki? You know, four acres is enough to make a life."

Then she takes Maddie Mae by the hand and the two of them leave me alone in the garden, stunned and finally understanding that all of this, all along, was for me.

FORTY-FOUR

Luella

We lost the forested South Carolina side of the kingdom and half the North Carolina side, but we regained our homes, and I was back in the kingdom by Christmas. Some of the residents returned, others didn't. Jola came back, along with her brother's family. And to my utter joy, Vernon and Sunny gave up the rented property and took up residence in the kingdom.

Wade still walked with a limp, and his eyes was too sad for such a young man, but he found joy on the kingdom land. I planned to celebrate his eighteenth birthday with a gathering in the yard. All the remaining kingdomfolk would be invited.

Sunny was now carrying a child. Them first few months was difficult for her, so I helped with the mending she took in. I still didn't like the needle, but all of us sometimes had to do work that didn't bring joy. That was just the way of our lives.

By summer of the following year, the kingdom was back to life, though different than before. We didn't have children for the schoolhouse, but there was a chicken coop, a corncrib, and a barn.

William slept in the house down the lane, close enough where we could get to him if he needed us. Robert opened a shoe shop. Me and Jola used the cart to deliver flowers. My business was good so I had to expand my garden. Wade and his friends helped, though Wade took a job in town. When I asked him what he planned to do, he told me he wanted to study under a barber. It saddened me that the labor camp had all but stamped out my boy's love of the outdoors, but I understood. We hadn't had a choice during slavery. Working inside or outside was decided for us. This was one of the pleasures of freedom. Wade could cut hair all year round and didn't have to work in that old dusty mill if he didn't want to. He could work free of the rain on his back or the snow in his boot. He could dress like a gentleman to go to work.

Sunny's baby was born that summer, and they named him William. She had been scared to share her choice with us, afraid Robert might get jealous. But all we felt was joy when William held the baby in his hands for the first time and kept saying over and over, *William? That's his name? Sure enough? William?*

The wound between the brothers was healed enough for Robert to tease his brother. *You stole my own children right out from under me and now you got my first grandchild!* And the two of them laughed. We had become a family of two fathers, two grandfathers, brothers bound by the crooked life we'd found in these hills.

It was not lost on me that I loved them both. When I looked at the two brothers, I no longer compared them like I used to. I saw two different men who had been there for me in all the right ways and was grown enough to admit when they hadn't. They was the Montgomery brothers, but they was also Robert and William, my two men. Robert, my lover. William, my friend. And I wouldn't have it no other way.

341

Every now and then, I walked the property by myself just to sit with my memories. I closed my eyes and remembered the hill of purple flowers that smelled like heaven, the morning sounds of the settlement coming to life as the women rose to cook the morning meal, the sound of the drum to herald the birth of a baby. I remembered how the council had sat together when the moon shone bright in the sky, discussing our futures with all the enthusiasm of the newly rebirthed.

Then I'd turn around and walk the path back to the palace, carrying the hope that my children and my children's children would make something even better, that they'd carry with them the memory that we had tried our best to give them something like home.

EPILOGUE

In spring, we welcome eighty-five kingdom descendants to our property. Eighty-five! I meet cousins I didn't know existed. Everyone pays dues, and those dues purchase food, T-shirts, and a tent to shield us from the mountain sun. Bryan is on program to deliver a presentation on Black genealogy, encouraging everyone to develop family trees for both sides of their families. I glance over at him.

There is power in knowing, he tells them.

I am the one tasked with telling the story of the kingdom, and though I'm nervous, I know I must begin with the story of Mother Rita, who fought until her last days to hold on to our family land. When I stand before them, it is as if the wind carries my breath, a song from the ancestors on my tongue.

My grandmother made it to Christmas and then passed quietly in her sleep just before the new year. When I went to wake her for our morning walk, I knew when I opened the door that she had transitioned. I was calm as I made the necessary calls. Then I lay beside her on the bed and wrapped an arm around her, inhaling the rose scent in her hair.

Dearest kingdom family. I come to you today with a story that will sound impossible to your ears, but that is as real as the ground on which you plant your feet. Touch this ground. Feel this soil. And know that on one late summer day in 1873 your ancestors walked up this mountain all the way from Cross Anchor, South Carolina, to create a better life for themselves.

From the corner of my eye, I can see Mama watching me, pride written across her face. In the back, R.J. sits between Shawnie and Maddie Mae, who sits in the seat Mother Rita would have occupied. Though Maddie isn't a kingdom descendant, we all wanted her here on this day to represent her best friend.

Shawnie smiles at me. Inspired by her newfound knowledge that Lily Lovejoy was a teacher, she says she wants to teach, too. She has applied to Bennett College in Greensboro and is waiting to hear if she was accepted.

They called it the Kingdom of the Happy Land. And Luella Montgomery, along with her husband William and her second husband, Robert, were declared the king and queen. The kingdom dwellers established a communal treasury, and they were able to save and purchase the land. Two hundred acres of God's country right here in North Carolina, roughly half of which was in Luella's name and the other in Robert's name. They were landowners, governors of their own bodies, caretakers of their futures. They did that so we could come here today and gather in their name. Freedmen and women, children of God.

I hold up the water pitcher I found in the palace, a pitcher I believe dates all the way back to the kingdom. As they pass it around, I look out over my friends and family. Nearly a hundred and fifty years prior to my conception, Luella fought to save the land for her family so they could have a place to call home. Now we have been able to do the same. Together, the women of this family have saved this land and legacy, used our smarts to keep us here on this mountain that has given us refuge. I didn't think we could do it, but we did. We were only able to save four acres, but it is enough. More than enough. Now our entire family will be stewards of this place once again, will understand this rootedness is a gift. When we call ourselves kings and queens, it isn't just a fantasy of Black pride. It means something.

I am the descendant of a queen, a real queen, and I guess that makes me one, too.

MAMA HOLDS MY hand tightly as we walk down the path, the springtime breeze on our faces.

"Mother Rita would've loved the gathering," I say. "She would've held court."

"Yes, she would have. But she was there. Everybody buried in that cemetery was there."

I believe that, too. The spirits of my people still roam the kingdom and walk the land. They stand nearby, watching us.

"You didn't forget the sketch, did you?"

I shake my head.

In the distance, just over the hill, is Albert's house. I wonder what Jessica is doing with the boys this summer, if they are in camp or if they're still begging to play video games all day. I had fondue with her and her friends the week before. It was fun, though there was an awkward moment when her husband passed through the living room.

When we arrive at the graveyard, Mama places the canvas bag on the ground. I spread the map on the grass and place a book on it so it won't blow away. We take the little handwritten signs and stick them in front of the rocks as Mother Rita instructed.

"They said the stones will arrive in a few months. I hope we have all the name spellings correct."

"I'm sure we won't have them perfect. Sometimes they vary among census takers," I say. I've been learning more about census records in my research. I give her a little smile, as if to apologize for sounding like I know so much. But Mama just says, "Isn't that something? I never looked in those records."

"I can show you, if you'd like. I've looked through those websites so many times, I'm probably an expert by now."

"I'd like that."

We continue to put the markers in their correct places, pushing the stakes down low enough that they won't become uprooted by heavy rains.

I pause for a moment. "I have a question for you, Mama."

She rises up slowly. "Anything. Ask me anything."

"Mother Rita once said she named me. Is there any truth to that? Is that why she always called me by my birth name, Veronica?"

"Let's finish up here, and I'll show you something."

Once all the stakes are placed, we gather our belongings and walk up the hill, away from Mother Rita's house. Though I'd easily gotten lost while chasing a bird that day, Mama looks comfortable on the land, as if she has never forgotten it. She wears my binoculars around her neck, and every now and then she brings them to her eyes, though she doesn't share with me what she is spotting. I don't mind the silence. I just want to walk with her for a bit.

I remember some of the things Mother Rita taught me. *Zinnia seeds can be scattered or they can be sowed into the soil about a quarter inch from the surface. The leaves are large and green and hardy, but they can be hard to weed and will take over a garden if you're not careful. Deadhead them because it'll make the stems even longer and the blooms more frequent.*

I have found something on this land I never knew I needed. There is something about being out here that makes me feel renewed and content. I'm still scared of snakes, but I love this place. It's yet another newly discovered part of myself.

Keep your scissors sharp, and when they become dull, sharpen them the old-fashioned way on a strop. Some of the blooms love to be cut at sunrise when the dew is still fresh on the ground. Drop the stem in a bucket of water with flower food. They can stay in that bucket for twelve to twenty-four hours without wilting one bit.

We come out of the woods at the top of a ridge and Mama points. I look out over a field of conelike purple flowers shooting out of green stems. Bees rise and hover over the tall, spiky flowers, as if guarding the field while also feasting upon it. "What is all this? Lavender?"

"It's a kind of lavender. It's also known as speedwell, but Mother Rita called it by its proper name. *Veronica.*"

"I'm named after a flower?"

"Yes, you are."

I look out over the flowers, standing so tall they waver in the breeze.

"This was Mother Rita's happy place. When she was younger, she'd even bring a folding chair and a book. When I named you

Veronica, it was like a quiet signal to her that I still loved her. I suppose she considered your name her legacy."

I step forward, away from Mama, as if to step into my new self once more. I have been making these moves over and over again for the past year. I am now forty years old, and I'm learning new things about myself each day. I had a late start, but there is time to make it up.

Beneath that sun, I make a promise to myself. If I'm fortunate enough to be granted more time on this earth, I will read more books. I will plant lots of flowers. I will be the great-great-great-granddaughter of Queen Luella's dreams.

In this field, once tended by men and women stepping out of their past and into their future, I will seek the footsteps they left behind and I will walk in them.

AUTHOR'S NOTE

In fall of 1873, a group of freedpeople left Spartanburg County, South Carolina, headed north across the state line into North Carolina. Near Zirconia, North Carolina, the people established a remote community that they called a kingdom. They named a king and queen, formed a communal treasury, and eventually purchased 205 acres of land in 1882 from John Davis, land that was spread across the North Carolina–South Carolina state line. Approximately half was deeded to Luella Montgomery and the other half to Robert Montgomery.

At its height, it is believed the kingdom numbered over two hundred people. By the turn of the century, the kingdom began to decline in numbers, though some of the acreage stayed in the possession of kingdom descendants until 1919, when it was finally sold.

Sadie Smathers Patton, a Henderson County historian, published a pamphlet in 1957 that has long been considered the definitive resource on the kingdom. Journalists and academics alike have cited this pamphlet as a primary source. Based on Patton's information, the freedpeople walked north from Mississippi, seeking new life after slavery ended.

However, I have not found any evidence that the original kingdom dwellers were from Mississippi. I believe they originated from Cross Anchor, South Carolina, driven out of Spartanburg County under the threat of terrorist violence.

Over the years, the kingdom's existence has been corroborated by field researchers and kingdom descendants. Many of the details of the kingdom in this novel are inspired by newly discovered facts from the archives, though I admit I have taken liberties, as any good storyteller must.

In my imagining of the kingdom, it is both a literal and metaphorical manifestation of a people's desire to rise into their full humanity. As a native Southerner, I understand this deep connection between a community and the land they inhabit. This relationship to the land is fundamental to how we Southerners view ourselves.

As I considered the story I wanted to tell about the kingdom, I couldn't help but be deeply moved by their tenacious desire for land ownership and self-sufficiency. This history of African American industriousness is often overshadowed by what followed. Though they did not ultimately lose the kingdom land by nefarious means, a lot of African Americans did. Using Census of Agriculture data, scholars conservatively estimate that African Americans lost $326 billion in land wealth between 1910 and 1997. I was stunned by the magnitude of this loss and its continued impact on racial economic disparity in the United States. There was no way I could tell this story of the kingdom without connecting it to its full context.

Heirs' property loss continues to this day. There is remarkable work happening at the state level to ensure families are protected from this injustice. I have been inspired by the work of legal scholar and 2020 MacArthur Genius Grant recipient Thomas W. Mitchell, the primary architect of the Uniform Partition of Heirs Property Act (UPHPA), a legislation that helps close the legal loophole of land loss among rural American families by ensuring there is due process. As of now, twenty-four states have enacted the legislation and six have introduced it.

At the time of this book's publication, North Carolina has introduced the legislation, but has not passed it.

If you want to follow the states (including your own) that are introducing and enacting this legislation, you can view the map at uniformlaws.org. If you want to learn more about the Kingdom of the Happy Land, you can visit the link at my website: dolenperkins valdez.com.

The freedpeople who established the Kingdom of the Happy Land were not unlike millions of people who dreamed of land ownership, standing firm in their belief that property was the surest path to full citizenship and the benefits therein.

Oh, how they dreamed! Oh, how they imagined!

ACKNOWLEDGMENTS

My heart of hearts is and always will be my mom. If you have ever met my mom, you know that she is a dynamic force. If I have done anything good in this world, it's because she taught me empathy. If I have written any memorable characters, it's because she taught me to listen when people are speaking. So many of the creative women of my mom's generation didn't have the opportunities to write books, paint sunsets, and compose music. Instead, they supported us, their children. I honor all those women. And I honor you, Mom, a brilliant writer and artist in your own right. Thank you for everything, BP.

When I first discovered the Happy Land in 2022, I reached out to Ronnie Pepper, librarian at Henderson County Public Library and oral storyteller who has been working to keep the story of the kingdom alive through community events. After our phone chat, I booked a flight to Hendersonville, North Carolina, to meet Ronnie in person, and during that trip he introduced me to Suzanne Hale, a friend who was interested in historic preservation.

ACKNOWLEDGMENTS

The three of us bonded over our curiosity about the kingdom, and, during a delectable dinner prepared by Suzanne (who I would later learn is a retired international diplomat and ambassador), I had a feeling our little trio would turn out to be magical.

And I was right.

Suzanne was brilliant at sifting through the local archives for little-known historical documents. Ronnie's insight and wisdom proved invaluable when our paper trail hit a dead end. Ultimately, the three of us uncovered history that no one has ever documented. I am so grateful to Suzanne and Ronnie, who have taught me that part of writing a book is making lifelong friends along the way. Also, thanks to David Payne for allowing me to tour the property that was originally owned by the kingdom.

Darrick Hamilton, the Henry Cohen Professor of Economics and Urban Policy at the New School, patiently answered my questions about heirs' property. Mavis Gragg, CEO of HeirShares and current Loeb Fellow at Harvard, provided the perspective of a seasoned lawyer and native North Carolinian. Willie Heyward, an heirs' property lawyer based in Charleston, South Carolina, helped ground me in the early months of my research. Cheryl Kurss, my longtime real estate agent and friend in Washington, D.C., answered questions about adverse possession.

I teach creative writing at American University in Washington, D.C., and I have the most amazing students. Three of my former graduate students—Alexis Bland, Thaer Husien, and Faith Angel Campbell—were absolutely invaluable resources. My colleague Professor Jessica Waters always takes my calls. Our conversations enrich me. I am grateful to the university for the much-needed sabbatical it took to finish this book.

I have pored through countless sources trying to find a possible recipe for the Happy Land liniment. I have read about Reconstruction-era violence and the 1871–72 KKK trials in South Carolina. I have visited Cross Anchor, the home of the original Happy Land settlers; perused newspapers; cold-called people who never responded; scanned maps; toured flower farms; and studied legal documents. One of the reasons I appreciate historical fiction so much is that I understand the work that goes into writing a novel such as this one. So I take this moment to send a grateful shout-out to all the folks who read and write and love historical fiction. You are amazing! I appreciate you so much. (Also, if you love historical fiction as much as I do, you can join my online book club on my website.)

Some wonderful writers offered words of support for my previous book *Take My Hand*: Celeste Ng; Kate Quinn; Terry McMillan; Robert Jones, Jr.; Christina Baker Kline; Chris Bohjalian; Nicole Dennis-Benn; Fiona Davis; Jamie Ford; Stephanie Dray; and Victoria Christopher Murray. Also, a special message of gratitude and love to the late novelist, journalist, and mentor to so many Tina McElroy Ansa.

Thank you to my dream team at Berkley Books, with a special shout-out to my indefatigable editor, Amanda Bergeron. I could not have done this book without you, Amanda. Truly. I can't wait for William and Madeline to do their promotional shoot! Francesca Main at Phoenix Books / Orion in the UK was also invaluable, and I am so grateful. My agent, Stephanie Cabot, is the best in the business. On top of that, she is my dear and forever friend.

My friends and family sustained me in the long months and years of writing this book. My brother, Harry, reminds me to slow down and cherish the small things in life. My niece, Barbara, and nephews, Stephen and Ross, are as close to me as my own children.

ACKNOWLEDGMENTS

The elders of my family—aunts Agnes, Carole, and Beverly and Uncle David—inspire me every single day. My in-laws, Rhina and Ovidio, wrap me in love. My friends are always the first to support my books, especially my longtime friend Leslie Lewis, who not only shouts out my books from the rooftops but never fails every single year to text at midnight on my birthday. My longtime friend Milton Brown is always there for me, and I'm so grateful for him. My daughters support me in so many ways. Elena walks the dog and brings me hot tea. Emilia makes colorful "do not disturb" signs for my door and organizes my desk. I am so grateful they understand that time with the book is time well spent.

And David. Well, what can I say to capture all that you do for me each and every day? You are the Virgo to my Gemini, the moon to my sun, my William and my Robert.

ABOUT THE AUTHOR

Dolen Perkins-Valdez is the *New York Times* bestselling author of three previous novels. Her most recent, *Take My Hand*, was nominated for multiple awards and selected for the BBC2 Between the Covers book club. She is an Associate Professor at American University and lives in Washington, DC with her family.